25 ESSENTIAL SKILLS for the Successful Behavior Analyst

This second edition of Bailey and Burch's best-selling *25 Essential Skills for the Successful Behavior Analyst* is an invaluable guide to the professional skills required in the rapidly growing field of applied behavior analysis.

The demands on professional behavior analysts, BCBAs and BCBA-Ds, are constantly increasing such that several new skills are required to keep up with new developments. Each chapter has been thoroughly updated and seven new chapters address recognizing the need to understand client advocacy, cultural responsiveness, and the movement toward diversity, equity, and inclusion in the field.

The authors present five basic skills and strategy areas which each behavior analyst need to acquire: essential professional skills, basic behavioral repertoire, applying behavioral knowledge, vital work habits, and advanced skills. This book is organized around those five areas, with a total of 25 specific skills presented within those topics.

Jon S. Bailey, PhD, BCBA-D, Emeritus Professor of Psychology at Florida State University for over 50-years, teaches ethics and professional issues graduate courses. Dr. Bailey was a founding Director of the Behavior Analyst Certification Board® and is past president of the Florida Association for Behavior Analysis.

Mary R. Burch, PhD, BCBA-D, is a Board Certified Behavior Analyst®. Dr. Burch has more than thirty years of experience in developmental disabilities. She has been a Behavior Specialist, QMRP, unit Director, and Consulting Behavior Analyst in developmental disabilities, mental health, and preschool settings.

"The skills described in this invaluable resource book are generic, that is they are relevant for virtually all professional endeavors. Uniting practice of them with knowledge of behavior analysis would supply behavior analysts an advantage in any field they chose to enter."

—**Patrick C. Friman, Ph.D.**, ABPP; Vice President of Behavioral Health, Boys Town; Clinical Professor of Pediatrics, UNMC

"This book provides precious direction on how to develop a robust set of professional skills. Among the recommended texts for new and practicing behavior analysts, this book stands as most important to me."

—**Martin Myers, BCBA**; President, Flatrock Advising; Editor, Flatrock Weekly

25 ESSENTIAL SKILLS for the Successful Behavior Analyst

From Graduate School to Chief Executive Officer

Second Edition

Jon S. Bailey and Mary R. Burch

Routledge
Taylor & Francis Group
NEW YORK AND LONDON

Designed cover image: Cover Design by CuneoCreative.com

Second edition published 2023
by Routledge
605 Third Avenue, New York, NY 10158

and by Routledge
4 Park Square, Milton Park, Abingdon, Oxon, OX14 4RN

Routledge is an imprint of the Taylor & Francis Group, an informa business

[First edition published by Routledge 2009]

ISBN: 978-1-032-20856-5 (hbk)
ISBN: 978-1-032-19207-9 (pbk)
ISBN: 978-1-003-26557-3 (ebk)

DOI: 10.4324/9781003265573

Typeset in Minion Pro
by Apex CoVantage, LLC

For Product Safety Concerns and Information please contact our EU representative:
GPSR@taylorandfrancis.com
Taylor & Francis Verlag GmbH, Kaufingerstraße 24, 80331 München, Germany

This 2nd edition of our *25 Essential Skills* book is dedicated to the memory of my former student and colleague of 40 years, Maxin Reiss, PhD, BCBA-D (1948–2018). You epitomized the necessary repertoire for successful behavior analysts and modelled it for our graduate students. You were instrumental in encouraging me to put this vision into print. I think you would be proud of the enhancements to your original model.

—Jon S. Bailey, BCBA-D

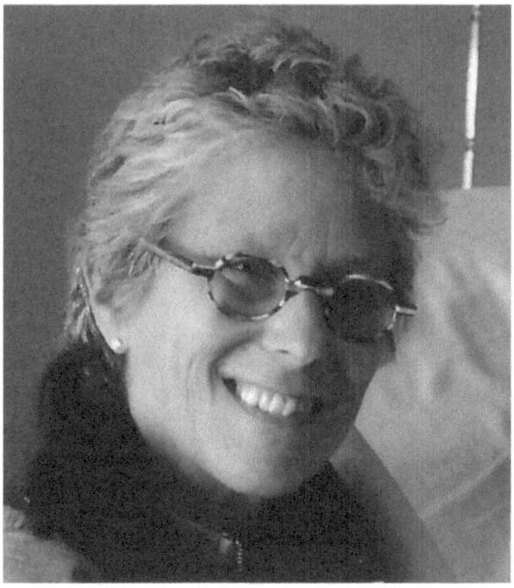

Figures

Preface to the 1st Edition

> I come home from working at the Developmental Disabilities Center twice a week, drop on the couch, and just cry. I don't know what's wrong with me. I think they just don't like me and don't trust me. I feel like an outsider. I have clients whom I love, and I enjoy the challenge of solving problems. I'm well paid by my consulting firm, but at the DD center they don't respect me, and they won't listen to me. I've been told the administrator talks about me behind my back. They like to use drugs for treatment instead of my behavior plans . . . . I can't admit to my supervisor that I'm in trouble. I don't know what to do, really, I don't. I'm board-certified, and I've taken Dr. Bailey's ethics course, but it's not helping me in this situation.

This emotional and heart-wrenching plea came to us in the form of a desperate phone call from Kimberly, a newly certified behavior analyst. This extremely bright, enthusiastic, go-getting graduate student had such an intense desire to get her first job and begin helping clients with behavioral needs that no one would have predicted she would find herself in the depressing situation she described. But she did.

We began to notice that many other behavior analysts were experiencing similar problems, and we had a revelation—being an expert in behavior analysis is *not* sufficient for a behavior analyst to be a successful consultant. As our field continues to grow, it is critical that we educate behavior analysts on *all* the skills needed to be effective and make a difference in the life of others.

Applied behavior analysis evolved from the experimental analysis of behavior in the mid-1960s. Our field became formalized in 1968 with the publication of the first issue of the *Journal of Applied Behavior Analysis* under the editorship of Mont Wolf at the University of Kansas. The blueprint for the field was established in a seminal article in that issue, "Some Current Dimensions of Applied Behavior Analysis," authored by Don Baer, Mont Wolf, and Todd Risley (1968). In this article, they outlined the key distinctions of this new field that made it different from the rest of psychology. As described in the article, behavior analysts were interested in solving applied problems by using a to-be-developed technology based on the science of behavior; that is, operant conditioning. This technology would be inherently data-based. It would its own methodology for demonstrating cause-effect, that is, the single-subject research design, and it would evolve over time to give us a vast array of techniques that would show how these procedures would help people improve the quality of their life. In 1968, the cutting-edge thought-leaders who authored this important article did not anticipate today's overwhelming demand for behavior analysis. This enormous need for services has developed in the past five years, and services are now provided in many countries by Board Certified Behavior Analysts®.

As a result, master's degree programs have sprouted like wildflowers across the United States and indeed the world. Two-year and three-year graduate programs that turn out behavior analysts by the hundreds are now working overtime to provide professionals to work with individual clients who are autistic, developmentally delayed, brain injured, or otherwise disabled. In some cases, behavior analysts are working one-on-one with clients, and in other situations, they are working with teams of paraprofessionals who are implementing behavior programs designed by a behavior analyst.

Behavior analysts are also working in business, industry, government, and organizational settings to improve human performance in safety-related areas or to increase productivity, product quality, or service. In these settings, the behavior analyst takes on the role of the consultant, the professional advice giver who must know a great deal about how organizations work and don't work and about how to train, motivate, and manage people in settings that were never designed from the outset to be optimal for human performance.

As it turns out, being an expert in behavior analysis does not provide all the necessary skills to be an effective, successful consultant. The settings where we work have often been visited before by other consultants who had no behavioral training whatsoever but who, with their finely tuned sense of business etiquette, social skills, and gift of gab, have made it difficult for the behavior-technology-savvy behavior analyst to make much headway. Upper-level management of human-service organizations and CEOs of major corporations now have an expectation of a quality of interaction that is hard to acquire in graduate programs that offer only courses in applied operant conditioning, research methodology, functional analysis, data collection, and practicum experience working one-on-one with an autistic child. And it turns out that working as a consultant in a developmental training center, in a classroom for children with behavior disorders, or with parents who need to learn how to manage their unruly children requires that the behavior analyst must interface with a wide variety of people who present (a medical term meaning "show up with") an amazing array of contentious and obstructive behaviors that can thwart the unwary and unprepared would-be behavioral consultant.

This became obvious when the first author was contacted by the supervisor of a recent graduate—a hardworking and bright individual who was failing on one of his first consulting assignments. This budding behavior analyst was yet another young professional who found himself in a dilemma much like the one Kimberly described to us (in the case at the beginning of this preface). According to the supervisor, the new behavior analyst had missed the initial cues from management that he was in trouble, and when he finally learned there were problems, he did not seek help. His tendency was to blame the direct-care staff for their shortcomings and failure to carry out his programs. Upon further investigation, he had simply been unprepared for a semi-hostile school environment that paid lip service to wanting behavioral consultation but in truth was set in its traditional ways.

Rather than rebuke or blame the new consultant, the first author made an attempt to determine what went wrong in his training. This led to countless interviews with current and former students, supervisors of consultants, trainers of consultants, and CEOs of companies that hired behavior analysts. In addition, senior consultants were asked a series of questions about their experiences dealing with tough problems in a variety of settings, how they solved these problems, and what they had learned from the experience. When possible, these consultants and supervisors were asked to provide working scenarios that described in a concise format the nature of the problems encountered.

From these interviews and written scenarios, we developed over a six-month period key words and descriptors of skills and strategies. At this stage, about 100 descriptive terms emerged as important skills and strategies for successful behavior analysts. This number of skills was clearly too many to try to describe or teach. We began a search of sources of knowledge that might prepare the consultant in training for the difficult road ahead. Using key words and Amazon.com, we found it was possible to determine recent books that seemed to focus on the key skills we identified, even though they were not specifically written for our new type of professional: the behavior analyst consultant. Although these books were written for professionals in other fields, it was clear that they had relevance for us. They denoted and described general categories that are clearly required for any professional operating in someone else's setting; topics such as business etiquette, assertiveness, and leadership were common. We found that the business consulting literature emphasized that professionals should have excellent personal communication and persuasion skills as well as a strong background in negotiation, lobbying, and public speaking. As categories of skills and strategies that began to encompass our original list of 100 emerged, a solution to the problem of categorizing our comprehensive list of required skills began to look possible. By reanalyzing the scenarios that we had gathered in terms of "What skills would it take to fix this?" we eventually were able to formulate five general categories of skills and strategies. In addition to having the basic skills just described, consultants would have to be prepared to apply their knowledge of behavior analysis to deal with what is known in the business literature as "difficult people." The good behavior analyst must know how to use his or her knowledge of functional analysis, shaping, and performance management to deal with these problems and ask pointed questions about issues that come up daily with "Can I see that?"

As a professional, the behavior analyst must also confront the difficult task of managing his or her own behavior on a daily basis. Without careful monitoring, even bright, highly motivated behavioral consultants can waste time, be a burden to other professionals, get stressed out, and find themselves needing help but not knowing how to go about getting it.

One final area emerged from our interviews and scenario collection. There is an expectation that behavioral consultants will grow over time, roughly a five-to-seven-year period when they are expected to take senior consultant positions. These positions will involve additional responsibility, and the need for greater wisdom in making decisions can have a wide-ranging impact on the organizations served. From preschools to factories, experience teaches consultants to refine their critical-thinking skills and to anticipate and quickly troubleshoot problems that invariably arise while consulting in any setting. Senior consultants are expected to take on training, coaching, and mentoring roles with newly minted behavior analysts and may engage in these important tasks with mid- and upper-level managers as well.

Finally, with time and experience, advanced consultants are expected to begin to see the "big picture" of how the world works and to develop an appreciation for the larger metacontingencies that control our society and our nation. This big picture analysis then expands to a broader worldview in which the consultant can suddenly begin to see the behavioral connections between his or her failed efforts to persuade a school principal to adopt a new discipline policy and the failure of an emergency relief effort in Myanmar.

The consultant who has developed advanced skills will have developed one of the most important skills of all—aggressive curiosity. Aggressive curiosity is the skill and attitude about the science of behavior that will enable the advanced consultant to see the beauty in measurement techniques that are robust enough to document the behavior problems of a client with Prader-Willi syndrome who routinely goes AWOL, track the cell phone usage of people in third-world countries, or monitor the feeding patterns of Antarctic penguins.

For the modern-day behavior analysis consultant, being competent and well trained in the technical aspects of behavior analysis is simply not enough. To be successful and effective, behavior analysis consultants need knowledge in critical areas of competence, which now also include essential business skills, basic consulting repertoire, the ability to apply behavioral knowledge, vital work habits, and advanced consulting skills.

25 Essential Skills & Strategies for the Successful Behavior Analyst was designed to be used as a companion to our book *Ethics for Behavior Analysts* (Lawrence Erlbaum Associates, 2005), in courses addressing ethics and professional issues in behavior analysis, or as a handbook for practicum courses where students are acquiring and testing their consulting skills for the first time. Supervisors of newly hired behavior analysts who consult in school systems, in residential facilities, or with families should also find the taxonomy useful in spelling out what their expectations are for professional representation of the consulting firm. Finally, experienced consultants might find the references to the professional consulting literature and checklists of value in improving their own skills.

Behavioral consulting is largely the art of practicing the science of human behavior. We hope that this book conveys the excitement and challenges that face our new colleagues as they join our ranks as professional behavior analysts.

—Jon S. Bailey and Mary R. Burch
2010

Preface to the 2nd Edition

This 2nd edition of *25 Essential Skills . . .* is intended to introduce the reader to a wide range of professional attributes that are expected in today's complex, competitive behavior analysis environment. Largely considered *soft skills* this expansive repertoire is quite the opposite; it represents a set of expectations for the 21st-century behavior analyst who must deal with a full range of challenges across many dimensions, some personal and many organizational in nature. A modern-day behavior analyst is expected to understand not only the technical details of our rapidly changing technology but they should also have a complete mastery of what is known as "The White Book." (Cooper, Heron & Heward, 2020). They are also expected to keep up with a flood of complex methods and techniques emerging from 50+ years of research published in the *Journal of Applied Behavior Analysis* (having a subscription is *de rigueur*). BCBAs are expected to be critical thinkers when it comes to consideration of magical and outlandish treatments that pop up like mushrooms in the spring from caregivers and yet have the social skills to explain to families in plain, polite English why it would be a violation of their ethics code to be involved with them. Administrators looking to hire a Board Certified Behavior Analyst are looking for well-rounded individuals who are calm, mature, organized, thoughtful, caring and above all else effective in diagnosing behavior problems (what is the *function* of this behavior?) and then designing and implementing effective behavior change programs based on that information. Company owners desperately want to add to their team a person with leadership skills who they can count on to train young people to become behavior technicians and therapists and then to take responsibility for their supervision; this is a special skill in itself that as it turns out few people have and which requires months, even years, of practice in behavior shaping (aka BST), goal setting, diplomacy, and an even-handedness that is near impossible to master given all the other demands of the job.

In this 2nd edition, now named *25 Essential Skills for the Successful Behavior Analyst*, we endeavor to capture the flavor of this vast array of talents and abilities that are now obligatory. We know that they will not all be acquired during the short, standard two-year period of training that most BCBAs currently receive. Those five or six semesters are full of courses on the techniques of ABA as applied to a variety of populations and settings. What is generally missing is any sense of what is expected by our consumers in the way of an actual professional repertoire; this book aims to outline those skills that we believe will make a difference in broadening the expectations of what it means to be a *successful* professional. We have begun each Unit with a challenge that captures the scope of the skills to be presented.

As you might expect, techniques for overcoming such challenges are not taught in most grad programs. We should add that this book alone will not provide all the answers, rather we hope that by explicitly naming the skills and introducing the content and process you will be able to seek the kind of post-BCBA training and experience necessary to make you a respected member of the behavior analysis community. For faculty, we hope that they will be able to create at least some opportunities for their students to explore these areas of expertise and to acquire basic skills in professional etiquette, interpersonal communications, leadership, cultural responsiveness, and so on.

This edition of the *25 Skills* book is divided into five units starting with *Essential Professional Skills* and *The Basic Professional Repertoire.* We believe that the ten skills included in Units 1 and 2 should prepare most graduates for their first jobs, not with expertise but at least the fundamentals to make a difference when working with the public. Unit 3, *Applying Your Behavior Knowledge*, highlights five skills closely related to basic principles of behavior but which will require a certain stretch to attain such as managing difficult people, knowledge and sensitivity to diversity, equity, and inclusion and applying behavior analysis in business and industry and in schools. Unit 4 adds five more essential skills for a BCBA to be effective day to day including time management, networking, dealing with stress, and of course, public speaking. In the final section, Unit 5, we propose some skill areas that are rarely taught in graduate programs but are surely going to be essential if a behavior analyst is going to grow professionally over time. These include creative problem-solving, critical thinking, a new chapter on *Design Thinking*, and finally, one of our favorite topics, aggressive curiosity.

A unique feature of this 2nd edition is the addition in each chapter of three sections pertaining to the development of one's career over time. As suggested by Dr. Baker Wright in early interviews regarding our book proposal, we now realize that these 25 Skills are not just for the newly minted BCBA but rather represent a foundation for a full lifetime commitment to the profession of behavior analysis. In short, behavior analysts grow up and with more and more years of experience, they are expected to take on more and more important duties as a behavior analyst supervisor, director, and eventually perhaps as an owner or a CEO. As they advance through the ranks and build up credibility and responsibility, more is expected of them. We characterized this in an early title draft as *25 Skills for the Successful Behavior Analyst: From grad school to the C-suite* but were persuaded that the latter term might be unfamiliar to potential readers. We firmly believe that as behavior analysts move up the ladder from being fresh out of grad school, to their first job, to becoming a young professional (3–5 years), then mid-career (6–10 years), and finally becoming a senior behavior analyst, that applying these 25 skills will be useful for one's entire career. Each chapter is set up then to introduce the skill and describe it in some detail and then provide possible elaborations for each of the subsequent maturations in professional development.

We hope that you enjoy this 2nd edition as much as we have in envisioning this development and maturation of behavior analysis and that you will find it useful as a guide to professional growth over your entire 25–30-year career. We have high hopes for the future development of our field and wish you well in whatever career path you choose and look forward to seeing you at future professional conferences.

—Jon S. Bailey and Mary R. Burch
August 2022

REFERENCE

Cooper, J.O., Heron, T. E., & Heward, W. L. (2020). Applied Behavior Analysis. 3rd edition. Pearson Education, Inc.: Hoboken, NJ.

Acknowledgments

We would like to thank Baker Wright who has taken over the helm of BMC after Maxin Reiss's untimely death. In early discussions with him about our plans to revise the 25 Skills book his first comment was, "You know that this isn't just a book for grad students, I've assigned it to my staff including those BCBAs with several years' experience. I think you need to describe how you think these fundamental professional skills can be useful at any stage of a person's career." After giving it some thought, we agreed on four benchmark stages of a behavior analyst's career as described in the Preface to the Second Edition. Other colleagues looked at drafts of chapter titles and made great suggestions for additions and deletions: Missy Olive, Dawn Bailey, and Kim Lucker-Greene's input early on helped us formulate the ultimate chapter lineup. Former students, now successful professional behavior analysts, read drafts of chapters and offered suggestions for improvement: Kolton Sellers and Hope McNally, we thank you for your dedication to ABA and your time providing expert input. Thanks also go to Loren Eighmie, a former student who kindly shared her complex session schedules to illustrate the busy calendar that behavior analysts must manage.

Finally, I would like to thank Sinan Turnacioglu, MD for educating me about his groundbreaking *Floreo* virtual reality device that could revolutionize behavior analysis treatment, as well as Einar Ingvarsson, PhD Director of Clinical Services at Virginia Institute of Autism and Kathleen Kariel, BCBA, Clinical Director who were so kind as to share the first behavioral data using this device; this was a mind-expanding experience. Thank you.

Unit One

Essential Professional Skills

A BCBA-D who supervises newly graduated BCBAs at a large ABA firm was overheard to say to a colleague at a conference:

> Someone in my position needs to know what to watch for in new hires just out of grad school. They can *talk* about behavior, but still need mentoring, especially on specialty areas, and they need training on our company's procedures. Most of our new hires are articulate and enthusiastic, but they need practice communicating with parents and caregivers.
>
> Our new hires are well-trained in ethics related to the Code, but we see them needing coaching when it comes to their own ethics, as in, don't promise more than you can deliver and don't discuss clients with anyone else.

DOI: 10.4324/9781003265573-1

They usually understand "Think Function" related to clients, but they still need reminders about the function of stakeholder behaviors and especially their *own* behaviors.

But they are motivated and eager to learn. With good supervision, I feel that these new graduates will develop broader skills over time.

1

Professional Etiquette (Behaviors)

FRESH OUT OF GRAD SCHOOL, FIRST JOB

By the time you decide to pursue a career in behavior analysis, you will be aware of the many tasks that will come with your new job. Completing assessments, designing behavior programs, meeting with families, supervising RBTs, and evaluating client progress, are just a few of the behavior analytic skills you will need.

> Behavior analysts are in a rather intense competition with people in other professional services, and even though this has been the case for quite some time now, some behavior analysts might not be aware of this development.

In addition to these technical skills, there will be several other critical skills required for you to be successful in the behavior analytic workplace. One of these skill sets is *professional etiquette.* Professional etiquette is the way in which we conduct ourselves in a professional or business setting. Being polite and having good manners are the foundation of etiquette.

Key etiquette behaviors in the professional setting include using appropriate greetings and introductions, refraining from gossiping, demonstrating good manners during business meals

DOI: 10.4324/9781003265573-2

and events, listening, and not interrupting, turning off your cell phone during meetings and business meals, dressing appropriately for work, being punctual, communicating well (without jargon), using good eye-contact, and having a warm smile for most occasions.

Good etiquette also involves showing you are respectful and genuinely interested in others and remembering that please and thank you go a long way. Behavior analysts who have good professional etiquette skills create great first impressions by making others feel at ease. Your good etiquette leads to others thinking of you as likable, capable, and professional. Depending on the number of years you have been a behavior analyst, the etiquette skills related to you may vary.

Since graduate schools focus almost entirely on the science and technology of behavior analysis, little time is spent on the professional skills needed to effectively bring our talents to our consumers. As a field, behavior analysts have a long way to go in terms of our image. If we compare applied behavior analysis to premium professional services regarding how we present ourselves to our potential clients, there is often quite a contrast. Our "service representatives," Board Certified Behavior Analysts®, are often young people with a casual attitude and even more casual attire. They often address their professors on a first-name basis, and this casual demeanor extends to the cavalier use of behavioral jargon in conversations with consumers and other professionals. While not intentional, these behaviors can be off-putting.

Behavior analysts are in a rather intense competition with people in other professional services, and even though this has been the case for quite some time now, some behavior analysts might not be aware of this development. The greatest pressure seems to be, somewhat surprisingly, in autism treatment. This is somewhat difficult to believe because from an evidentiary perspective there is essentially no competition. No other treatment currently available has the breadth and depth of applied research showing reliable, clinically significant changes in behavior. Unfortunately, the image presented to the public—our potential consumers—by many representatives of our field is that of a gaggle of behavioral geeks who spout technical terms that sound somewhat ominous and threatening. For example, *control*, *reversal design*, *contingencies*, *manipulation*, and *intervention* do not sound particularly user-friendly. Furthermore, when used to describe how they might be used in treating a child with autism, these expressions can be downright alarming. A child with ASD symptoms is someone's precious son or daughter who they love dearly. What parent wants to hear a professional say, "We're going to extinguish Bradley's behavior"? Loving parents want us to help Bradley, not extinguish him.

Compare this with the smooth and soothing talk of the well-prepared, perfectly groomed, and seasoned competition, and you will see quite a contrast. To our credit, the next generation of behavior analysts is more highly trained and better prepared than any previous group. These behavior analysts are enthusiastic and technically skilled, have a clear focus on results, and they have the drive and tenacity to stick with a child. But as we'll repeat several times throughout this book, being technically competent alone is simply not enough for the behavior analysis *professional.*

First Impressions

First impressions do count, and the very first of the 25 professional skills that must be addressed is *etiquette*: the customary polite, respectful behaviors expected of someone in a particular profession. This includes all the behaviors ranging from arriving on time for every in-home appointment and introducing yourself properly to saying goodbye to the principal when leaving a school, and everything in between. Let's look at the specifics that make up contemporary professional etiquette.[1]

1. Dress Appropriately for the Circumstances

It is better to be slightly overdressed than underdressed. Never wear wrinkled, worn, dirty, stained, or faded clothing. Avoid headwear, shorts, jeans, sweats or athletic clothing, t-shirts, flip-flops, and athletic shoes. Never wear anything that fits too snugly, is low-cut, or otherwise revealing. Depending on your company's policy, facial piercings (e.g., nose rings, eyebrow rings, etc.) should be removed, and tattoos should be covered. The policies related to tattoos and facial hardware could vary based on your geographical location with cities generally being more liberal about this than rural areas. For most professional settings, "tats" and nose rings should not be obvious to consumers.

2. Introductions Should Be Somewhat Formal

This means clearly stating your first and last name, your title, and the company/agency that you represent. Smile sincerely while providing steady eye contact. In earlier years, the 3-second handshake was the standard requirement for an introduction, but because the COVID pandemic made us all more sensitive to the spread of viruses, handshakes are no longer needed in business settings. When leaving a residence or a meeting, end with a closing. "Thank you for meeting with me" or, "It was a pleasure meeting you" are good standbys.

3. Conversational Skills

Starting with good eye contact and letting the person be the center of attention, provide leading questions. Turn on your listening persona (active listening with "Uh-huh," smiles, and head nods are essential conditioned reinforcers to keep the person talking). Make sure that you have good posture: sit up straight, have your hands folded in front of you, have good eye contact, and don't fidget. When appropriate, ask questions related to the topic the person is discussing. Do not start talking about yourself. Use your Dale Carnegie tips (Carnegie, 1981) to make the person feel important and give them space to express their concerns.

4. Meeting Etiquette

To show respect to the person with whom you are meeting, confirm the meeting in advance, and show up *on time*. The saying "If you arrive at the time the meeting is to start, you are ten minutes late" will always be relevant. Be prepared with all your materials including a pen and writing pad and turn off your cell phone. All the previously described conversation etiquette is required for business meetings as well.

Grad School

While you are still in grad school you will have many opportunities to apply what you have learned in this chapter about professional etiquette. In your practicum placement where you are working to accrue your supervision hours, you will be meeting frequently with parents, other caregivers, teachers, and stakeholders both at your clinic and for in-home, at school meetings, and training sessions. For each of these, you can practice your skills and hopefully receive feedback from your supervisor. If you have an opportunity to sit in on a client intake, you will be able to observe how the interviewer handles the parents' questions and describes the potential behavior analysis treatment or intervention.

Job Interviews

Your first opportunity to test your newly acquired professional expertise will be in job interviews where your purpose is to not only gain information about the company or agency, but also to make that all-important good first impression. Confirming the meeting a day or two ahead, showing up a few minutes early, and giving a proper professional greeting should give you a good head start on this objective. Using your Dale Carnegie skills to let the person know you are interested in their company and their views on how you would fit in are essential elements of the interview. Even if you are not interested in the job, be sure to thank the person for their time and leave a good *last* impression.

Your New Job

For your new job, be sure to dress in a manner that is acceptable to leaders or supervisors in the setting where you will be working. In the corporate setting for performance management behavior analysts, business suits, dresses, pantsuits or business pants and blouses will most likely be the standard attire. The dress code for the corporate job will usually be described in the company's Employee Handbook.

For those behavior analysts who work in schools and therapeutic settings, make sure you are not violating the dress code for the agency in which you are working. For example, some schools prohibit staff from wearing open-toe shoes (sandals). Know the rules regarding the dress code in the settings where you are providing services. Although we generally say, "No jeans or t-shirts," there may be some situations in which a behavior analyst is expected to be in a sandbox or to play sports. In these cases, if you'll be attending a meeting later in the day, you should keep a change of clothes in your car. Don't show up to a high-level meeting and expect everyone to understand why you are dressed for the playground.

Acceptable attire for women in the day-to-day job as a behavior analyst includes what is generally referred to as "business casual" attire. Examples are business shirts, knit tops, blouses, sweaters (as opposed to a hoodie), blazers, jackets or sports coats, business casual slacks, skirts, and dresses. If your consulting firm has a polo-style shirt with the company logo, this is fine too.

Examples of unacceptable attire include suggestive, risqué, or revealing attire; clothing made of sheer or see-through fabrics; sweatshirts and T-shirts; athletic wear; stiletto heels; sundresses; crop tops; midriff tops; tube tops; tank tops; undershirts; flannels; miniskirts; halter tops and halter dresses; sweatpants; jeans; leggings/tights with no cover such as a skirt, etc.; cargo pocket pants and slacks; Lycra anything; nylon jogging suits; novelty buttons; baseball-style hats; gaudy jewelry; and similar items of casual attire that do not present a business-like appearance.[2] You might tend to think jeans and T-shirts are okay in settings such as preschool classrooms "because that is what the staff wears," but remember that you are trying to establish yourself as a professional, and "student threads" will not help you gain the respect and credibility you need.

For men, oxford cloth shirts, clean and pressed polo shirts, and blazers or sport coats with business casual khakis or slacks will usually be acceptable. Not acceptable are jeans, T-shirts, tennis shoes, and baggy pants with underwear showing. For men, it is usually expected that any facial hair will be neatly trimmed. For both sexes, a generally conservative appearance is strongly recommended.

For meetings and presentations, you'll want to step up your level of dress. For men, a jacket is recommended for important meetings, such as when meeting with the school principal or the client's physician. For women who are attending meetings where they need to have a presence, traditional business clothes should be worn rather than the daily company polo shirt and slacks that are worn when working with children.

YOUNG PROFESSIONAL (3–5 YEARS)

Having survived the first few years in your new job means that you have mastered basic etiquette. Now it is time to focus on a broader audience—your colleagues and other professionals. The book title says it all; *How to Win Friends & Influence People* (Carnegie, 1981) is a good challenge for you to accept. It will bring rewards to you personally and to your company in the form of better relationships with the other professionals practicing in our space. You will need friends who are occupational and physical therapists, social workers, and speech-language pathologists since you may need to make referrals to them on behalf of your clients. Ideally, they will refer their clients to your company if they encounter behavior issues that are out of their scope of practice. Some professionals in other areas might have developed a bias against behavior analysts from what they learned in grad school, from the internet, or possibly from a previous first-hand experience. Your job is to turn them around and prove that you are a caring professional who respects what they do, and you are prepared to be a team player on behalf of your clients.

MID-CAREER (6–10 YEARS)

Settling In or Moving Up?

At this point in your career, you will have achieved considerable experience and status. People in your company will be coming to you with questions and seeking your advice. This can be a comfortable period where you have overcome a lot of obstacles, mastered your craft, understand your clients, and are ready to settle in and enjoy the work without the uncertainty associated with being the "new kid on the block."

Some behavior analysts will take a different approach and use this mid-career period as a launch pad for bigger and better things.

Some behavior analysts will take a different approach and use this mid-career period as a launch pad for bigger and better things. You may look forward to mentoring junior professionals as you begin to look for leadership opportunities in your company. All of this will a require smooth and polished repertoire worthy of someone who is moving up professionally. Additional expectations are that you will attain visibility not only in your community but nationally. With your experience and expertise, you should be on committees of your state behavior analysis chapter, and you should be accepting regular invitations to participate on committees and study groups of ABAI (the Association for Behavior Analysis International). Traveling about the country and giving invited addresses will give you exposure to leaders in the field and numerous opportunities to practice your "meet and greet" protocols.

SENIOR BEHAVIOR ANALYST

If you stay with the same company for a decade or more and aspire to take on a big challenge, you will find yourself in the "C-suite." This means that you are either briefing executives or have a new title yourself. The occupants of this elite division of the company include the following: CEO (Chief Executive Officer), COO (Chief Operating Officer), CFO (Chief Financial Officer) or CIO (Chief Information Officer). These titles apply to larger companies that may have been created by private equity buy-outs of smaller ABA companies and may have hundreds of behavior analysts employed. If you are making a pitch or giving a presentation to these executives, certain customary rules apply:[3] 1) Make sure that you have done your research not only on your topic, but also on who will be in the presentation. Knowing the personal agenda of the key person makes all the difference. Remember that some of these executives may be business people who are not BCBA-Ds; 2) Start by introducing yourself and tell why you are there (it will be by invitation so mention this person's name); 3) Make it clear that you are the expert on the topic at hand and that you understand the problem that the CEO is dealing with or the financial issue being dealt with by the CFO; 4) Listen more than you talk, keep your presentation brief and show the value it will bring to the company. Be prepared to answer questions and make your answers as succinct as possible; don't waste their time; 5) If possible, try to get some commitment on your proposal before you leave the room; and 6) Be sure to thank the person that arranged for you to be there, and of course, thank the rest of "Chiefs" who are sitting around the table.

SUMMARY

This chapter describes the customary practices that behavior analysts must adopt to be successful in the four stages of their professional careers from grad student to senior behavior analyst. We start with basic concepts of etiquette including how to converse with clients without sounding mechanical and uncaring, which means using the common vernacular rather than our operant terminology. We discuss the importance of making a good first impression with caregivers, stakeholders, and others by adopting certain dress codes and the behaviors that go with meeting new potential customers in our field. Newly minted behavior analysts will find that knowing and using etiquette behaviors will be useful in interviewing for their first job and in interacting with their new colleagues at work. Young professionals will encounter different challenges as they deal with professionals from other fields, and they should adopt a friendly and cooperative demeanor. Mid-career behavior analysts need to adopt certain specific etiquette techniques to be successful in chairing meetings and making them run smoothly. Those who stay with the same company or make the jump to a larger organization may reach the top level of the corporate ladder where the demands are great for a "C-level" etiquette repertoire that is essential for success. Learning to think strategically and to attend to the bottom line are required for senior behavior analysts as well as participating in media training in preparation for representing the company.

NOTES

1 www.burbankusd.org/cms/lib/CA50000426/Centricity/Domain/254/Professional%20Etiquette%20updated.pdf accessed 11/11/21
2 This list was compiled from several human resources web sites for retail and professional settings.
3 www.inc.com/geoffrey-james/c-suite-advice-7-rules-for-meetings-with-top-execs.html

REFERENCE AND FOR FURTHER READING

Carnegie, D. (1981). *How to win friends & influence people.* New York: Pocket Books.

2

Interpersonal Communications

IT'S NOT WHAT YOU SAY, IT'S HOW YOU SAY IT

Effective interpersonal communication skills are essential for all behavior analysts. Defined as "an exchange of information between two or more people" (Wikipedia, 2021),[1] interpersonal communications can be verbal or nonverbal. Verbal communications involve talking such as in meetings, on phone calls to clients and other professionals, and while giving presentations. Nonverbal communications include body language and written communications such as emails and texts. It is important for behavior analysts to be cognizant of both their verbal and nonverbal communications. Rolling your eyes in a meeting is not generally a good idea, while head nodding is a positive way to indicate your approval. The tone of emails can help or hurt the writer, so anything put in writing and sent to others should be carefully reviewed before sending.

For behavior analysts, interpersonal communications will cut across several areas. There is a clear connection to assertiveness, leadership, networking, collaboration, and public speaking. When behavior analysts communicate effectively, there are several valuable outcomes including keeping employees and teams or departments engaged, reducing turnover, better management of behavior analysts who are working remotely, improved interdepartmental communication or communication among consultants, and increasing client satisfaction.

DOI: 10.4324/9781003265573-3

FRESH OUT OF GRAD SCHOOL, FIRST JOB

Although you may have taken a course in Skinner's *Verbal Behavior* (Skinner, 1957), this does not begin to touch the fundamentals of the applied and contemporary, evidence-based field of interpersonal communications. Graduate students are so wrapped up in acquiring the philosophy, ethics, methodology, and scientific language of behavior analysis that adapting that worldview and jargon for everyday use in dealing with clients and stakeholders is understandably overlooked. Your primary needs for communication are with your professors and supervisors and to a lesser extent your clients and their family members or teachers, school administrators, and other professional colleagues. Effectively communicating with these individuals will be your bread and butter the minute you take off your cap and gown. You will need to use your everyday language skills far more often than the operant terminology you so laboriously memorized a few months earlier. The stakes are quite high so in many respects, your knowledge of ABA and your ability to translate that applied science into successful adoption by your consumers becomes Job Number One.[2]

In addition, we suggest you independently begin by focusing on the *message planning* phase of the communication process (Dillard, 2015, pp. 63–74), which begins prior to the first interaction with a new client, teacher, supervisor, or colleague. This includes doing some homework ahead of time so you have some idea of the person's concerns, what their preferences are for types of interactions, and your goal for the meeting. It is obviously not possible to plan for every meeting, so part of your planning is to reflect on what has worked in the past (known as "canned plans") (Verderber, Macgeorge, Verderber, & Pruim, 2016, p. 7). Being able to think on your feet and pull up an illustrative clinical example or apt metaphor that suits the person and the occasion is a necessary skill that every behavior analyst needs to acquire and the sooner the better.

> Developing these macro interpersonal skills also entails developing a robust repertoire of "*behavioral flexibility.*"

YOUNG PROFESSIONAL (3–5 YEARS)

After you have been on your first job for a year or so, you should have settled in and started to accept some additional responsibilities that will require more advanced interpersonal skills. These include taking on new challenges of being responsible for supervisees, responding effectively to your new supervisor, handling more difficult client/stakeholder cases, and possibly becoming involved in basic company governance and policy issues. To take on these more complex matters you will need to expand your "micro-skills" into "*macro-skills.*" This entails longer sequences of messaging such as "connecting with others in conversation," "managing difficulties with others, and influencing others." Developing these macro interpersonal skills also entails developing a robust repertoire of "*behavioral flexibility*" (Verderber etcal., 2016, pp. 23–25), which requires reacting in a variety of ways depending on the circumstances. Rather than just giving advice to a parent or teacher, you would start with active listening, followed by a sincere stream of conditioned reinforcers e.g., "That's interesting, can you tell me more?" "How did that make you feel?" and "I totally understand what you went through . . ." and then if you feel that the person is ready you may then offer some advice or a solution to the problem. It is expected that as you grow as a professional you will take on these more complex behavioral situations including those described as follows.

> *Supervisees need two things: guidance and assurance.*

Supervisors

As a young professional, depending on the size of the company, you will probably have a supervisor in the form of the clinical director or possibly the agency CEO or owner. Dealing with supervisors represents a different kind of challenge. As a grad student, you probably became used to your supervisor approaching you regularly for observation and feedback sessions, but this changes dramatically when you move into your first job. Here you will primarily be evaluated on your outcomes, i.e., how well your supervisees are doing, whether there are any complaints coming in about your performance from clients or colleagues, and of course how you are contributing to the bottom line of the business (making your billable hours, bringing in new clients, proposing new initiatives). You should become accustomed to the naturally occurring reinforcers from the professional and business world, which can be somewhat scarce. If you want feedback, you will probably have to add a new interpersonal skill; subtly seeking it from your supervisor in such a way that you don't appear "needy," which is a liability in the business of behavior analysis, e.g., "I just wanted to bring you up to speed on how my two new supervisees are progressing." One thing that most employees, including behavior analysts, fail to recognize is that being a supervisor is a very difficult and often lonely job that is carried out in a virtual "reinforcement desert." You may find that using your interpersonal skills to demonstrate appreciation for your hard-working supervisor will pay off in their fuller awareness of what you do.

MID-CAREER (6–10 YEARS)

When you reach this stage of your career, you will have clearly earned years of valuable experience and developed competence in several specialty areas. You will have fine-tuned the art of assessing client needs and communicating with families and your behavior analyst therapy teams. That difficult acquisition phase of your interpersonal communications skills should be complete, and you are ready to tackle communications within your agency or company. There is a good chance that you will have advanced in your leadership role in the company, have seniority among the other BCBAs, and are now expected to contribute to the smooth running of day-to-day operations including sitting on company special committees, chairing management meetings, and serving as a mentor to younger behavior analysts. Since your interpersonal communications skills now come naturally to you, this is the time to determine how these principles can be infused into the fabric of the organization. Failures of communication arise when those at the top are unable to effectively relay their vision of the company to all employees and when those in direct contact with clients are unable to share their daily frustrations with middle and upper management. This can result in less-than-optimal client outcomes, wasted opportunities for employee advancement, squandered resources, and employee turnover. It will take an experienced behavior analyst to fully understand the communication needs of the organization and to be able to develop functional solutions.

SENIOR BEHAVIOR ANALYST

To advance the understanding and acceptance of ABA, it is important for each organization to become a reliable, respected partner in community social initiatives. The core values of the company should become apparent in the way that they become involved in community projects. As a senior behavior analyst with more than ten years' experience, you will be expected to put your interpersonal communications skills to good use as you help define your company's values and propose ways of supporting community-based initiatives. Using the practices of our evidence-based field, you may be able to offer ways of evaluating the effects of these initiatives and promoting the involvement of your employees in those that are the most effective.

SUMMARY

This chapter outlines the interpersonal communication skills that a behavior analyst needs to be successful at four stages of their career from graduate student to senior behavior analyst. These skills include message planning, active listening, attending to body language, providing regular verbal and body language reinforcement, and expanding micro skills into macro skills. Young professionals need to expand their skills to include behavioral flexibility. While interacting with others, behavioral flexibility makes it possible to react on the spot to changing circumstances. In ABA, the importance of interpersonal communication skills with a variety of individuals becomes critical.

NOTES

1 https://en.wikipedia.org/wiki/Interpersonal_communication 9.5.21
2 Many professionals who live by their verbal skills have found that Toastmasters International (www.toastmasters.org) is a valuable organization to join to fine tune their public speaking and business communications skills.

FOR FURTHER READING

Carnegie, D. (1981). *How to win friends and influence people*. New York: Simon & Schuster.

Dillard, J. P. (2015). Goals-plans-action theory of message production: Making influence messages. In D. Braithwaite & P. Schrodt (Eds.), *Engaging theories in interpersonal communication: Multiple perspectives* (pp. 63–74). Thousand Oaks, CA: Sage.

Verderber, K. S., Macgeorge, E. L., Verderber, R. F., & Pruim, D. E. (2016). *Interact: Interpersonal communication concepts, skills and contexts* (14th ed.). New York: Oxford University Press.

Wikipedia (2021). https://en.wikipedia.org/wiki/Interpersonal_communication

Wood, J. T. (2015). *Interpersonal communication: Everyday encounters* (8th ed.). Boston: Cengage Learning.

3

Ethics in ABA

In looking for people to hire, you look for three qualities: integrity, intelligence, and energy. And, if they don't have the first, the other two will kill you.

—Warren Buffett

FRESH OUT OF GRAD SCHOOL, FIRST JOB

Your New Job

To recent graduates on their first full-time jobs as BCBAs, keeping track of ethics code standards while managing client cases and supervising RBTs and BCaBAs can seem overwhelming, but it is a critical part of the job. Detecting an ethical problem is one thing but coming up with a solution is quite another. Issues related to ethical conduct may not have been evident when you were interviewed. These troubling issues sometimes first appear when you bring a problem to management and hit a wall. The company may have hired the father of one of the clients as the facility accountant and you may notice that his child seems to get preferential treatment compared to the other clients. This is the natural consequence of a dual relationship (some call it a multiple relationship) and by the Code, it needs to be resolved:

> Code 1.11 If multiple relationships arise, behavior analysts take appropriate steps to resolve them. When immediately resolving

DOI: 10.4324/9781003265573-4

> a multiple relationship is not possible, behavior analysts develop appropriate safeguards to identify and avoid conflicts of interest in compliance with the Code and develop a plan to eventually resolve the multiple relationship.

This will be a test to determine if your company or association is serious about supporting the Code of Ethics. If they cannot resolve it in an ethical manner, you will have your work cut out for you going forward. Other barriers to ethical treatment may come from other sources as well including a school district with their policies, families that are resistant to implementing behavior programs, and a lack of resources for providing the ethical treatment of clients.

Barriers to Ethical Conduct

It is in this period where the enthusiastic, idealistic, ethically minded behavior analyst may have an awakening regarding ethics. It could appear that there are barriers and limits to providing ethical treatment. One obvious fact is that doing the right thing takes resources. In some cases, the resources are time or funding, and, in many cases, it is just a matter of having adequate staff or special expertise. You may know the right thing to do to meet the requirement of evidence-based treatment (Code 2.01) but the money to pay for it is not there, you feel you could meet the client's needs if you only had 20 hours per week, or if you could only somehow get them to Kennedy Krieger Institute.[1] Code 2.19 says to "remove or minimize the conditions" that "prevent service delivery" but this may be beyond reach or an impossible task.

Unethical Conduct by Nonbehavioral Colleagues

Dealing with the ethical conduct of nonbehavioral colleagues presents a different sort of challenge because they are not required to subscribe to *our* Code of Ethics. And there is a very good chance that their profession does not have anywhere near the commitment that we do to data-based decision-making. The best advice is to make every attempt to establish a working relationship in the best interest of your client. If you have established yourself as a reinforcer for this nonbehavioral colleague, and if you have demonstrated that you are a person of integrity, you may be able to ask questions or begin a discussion about some actions you think are unethical. Choose your words carefully, be sure to start with some open-ended questions, and avoid direct accusations. It is possible that you are wrong or that you have misinterpreted some action. You do not want to offend this person. Ideally, you'll be able to bring her to see the situation the way you do. Your hope is that the result of your interactions will result in effective treatment for the client. One of the most important things to remember is to be respectful of other professionals. Listen, learn about their perspective, and make every attempt to work together to help the client.

Unethical Conduct by Behavioral Colleagues

As unusual as it seems, from time to time, colleagues who are behavior analysts will present challenges. For example, some behavior analysts work for an agency where there are ten or more Board Certified Behavior Analysts (BCBA) or Board Certified Assistant Behavior Analysts (BCaBA)®. These days, behavior analysts can have completely different backgrounds in terms of their training. Some of them may have taken their course work and practicum in a standard two to three-year graduate program with faculty specially prepared for the task. Others may have taken the bulk of their work online and then received their supervision hours later. The exposure to ethics training for both groups of behavior analysts could range from a few lectures to an entire 3-credit-hour course over a standard 15-week semester. If you were a graduate student who sweated in three classes a week for 15 weeks over scenario after scenario trying to figure out the most ethical solution to a complex problem, and then you had to defend your answer in front of your colleagues, you may be more sensitive to ethical dilemmas than a student who just listened to a lecturer on the computer. In any event, you should know that everyone does not take the task of worrying about ethical conduct as seriously as you might.

If you carefully study Ethics Code for Behavior Analysts, you will notice the standards cover the most frequently occurring situations you will encounter. If you work in the vicinity of other behavior analysts, you may see occasional violations of the Code, and you'll need to decide whether to act. The Code can provide you with some assistance because it directs you to "address concerns about the professional misconduct of others directly with them" (BACB Ethics Code p. 5). Where you draw the line on the ethical violation is not clearly spelled out, but the prior commitment to integrity suggests that it would not take a major infraction for you to respond. Because you may be dealing with a fellow employee, it is best to start with a simple, unaccusatory question about what you know or saw, then ask for a meeting, explain your concern, and look for a reaction. There is a good chance the person's response will satisfy you, and you can move on with your life. If you still have a concern that the person is presenting a threat to the client, the company, or the profession, you will need to let your conscience be your guide, because the Code does not specify further action on your part. Sometimes it will be a good idea to seek advice from your supervisor or the supervisor of the other person.

Right to Effective, Least Restrictive Treatment

The data-based treatment approach used in behavior analysis puts us in a unique position in relation to other human services. On an almost daily basis, the behavior analyst will be confronted with a decision on the most appropriate treatment for a client where the alternatives involve fad treatments, warmed-over placebo effects, or outright frauds being pushed as though wishful thinking and hope were all that mattered. In our field, we take a hard-line stance on such fly-by-night nostrums, potions, and elixirs, and our Code indicates that "When a behavior analyst is concerned that services concurrently delivered by another professional are negatively impacting the behavior-change intervention, the behavior analyst takes appropriate steps to review and address the issue with the other professional." (BACB Ethics Code 2.18 p. 12). As behavior analysts, we must ensure our treatments are grounded in peer-reviewed applied research (Bailey & Burch, 2018), and they must be constantly evaluated while the treatment is in place (BACB Ethics Code 2.18 p. 12). Our guidelines further specify that we avoid harmful reinforcers, recommend reinforcement instead of punishment, and eliminate those conditions that might hamper the proper implementation of behavior programs (BACB Ethics Code 2.19 p. 12). This latter guideline is an essential part of the ethical conduct of professionals in our field. Because we rely on mediators to carry out the programs we write, we need to make sure that they are qualified to do so. We also need to train them competently and monitor their performance.

Integrity

One of the most important challenges to the daily conduct of the professional behavior analyst is the integrity of the services provided (BACB Core Principle 3, 2020).[2] If we are to instill confidence in our consumers, it is essential that they come to see us as truthful, reliable sources of information about behavior and how it can be changed. Ethical behavior analysts do not promise what they cannot deliver, shade the truth, make outlandish claims, or waver from a commitment. They certainly *do* obey the law. Promises matter, and the extent to which a behavior analyst can consistently deliver exactly what was promised on time, and with no excuses, is the extent to which the behavior analyst will be seen as ethical. A person with integrity is one who cannot be persuaded to take a different position just because it is popular, easy, or even rewarding in some immediate way.

> **Ethical behavior analysts do not promise what they cannot deliver, shade the truth, make outlandish claims, or waver from a commitment.**

One current dilemma presents an excellent example of a challenge to the integrity of behavior analysis services, and that is the plethora of "alternative" therapies offered to parents of ASD children with autism spectrum disorder (ASD). Behavior analysts tell us they are asked almost daily by parents or stakeholders about Floortime, hyperbaric oxygen treatment, facilitated communication (FC)/Supported Typing, gluten-free and casein-free diets, sensory integration, auditory integration, and more. Parents want your opinion and often want you to tell them it is okay to engage the services of someone offering these non-evidence-based treatments. Our code of ethics says, however, that you must inform the client about our firm commitment to data-based approaches. *Integrity means upholding high moral principles*, and in this regard, we have three: (a) a responsibility to all parties affected by our services; (b) a commitment to evidence-based treatments; and, above all else, (c) do no harm.

Finding an Ethical Place to Work

When applying for that all-important first job, you will want to make sure that the agency where you are interviewing fully supports ethical business practices and the BACB Ethics Code for Behavior Analysts. See Chapter 14 in *Ethics for Behavior Analysts*, 4th edition for details on questions to ask during your interview (Bailey & Burch, 2022).

> After a few weeks on the job, it became clear to me the data that staff were turning in was made up. The supervisor denied there was a problem, and the administrator was no help at all.
>
> —Anonymous BCBA

The ethical dilemma "Anonymous" presented is a difficult one, but it must be resolved by some direct action on the part of the behavior analyst. The behavior analyst has an ethical responsibility to resolve the conflict and needed to deal directly with the administrator even if the outcome was not acceptable. We generally advise behavior analysts to take a copy of the Code with them to the meeting with the administrator and point out the items that are relevant. Most facilities receive state or federal funding and are subject to review on a regular basis. Knowingly operating on false information is a form of fraud that is punishable by fines and revocation of a facility's permit. A young, somewhat timid behavior analyst may not be willing to push the issue this far but would be right to do so including contacting the insurance company. The Code of Ethics for our field was specifically designed to provide support for professionals in the field who wish to protect clients' right to effective treatment.

YOUNG PROFESSIONAL (3–5 YEARS)

As you advance professionally in your organization, there will be an expectation that you will begin to support and develop the ethics of others who are your supervisees, trainees, and RBTs. A relevant standard is Code 1.01 *Being Truthful*. Given a concern in the field about reducing the potential biases among our personnel, there is one additional requirement described in Code 1.07, i.e., to "evaluate biases of their supervisees and trainees" so as to provide optimal behavioral support to "individuals with diverse needs" (BACB Ethics Code, 2020, p. 9). Developing training materials and methods to meet this objective is appropriate at this increased experience level.

MID-CAREER (6–10 YEARS)

As you reach the mid-career level, it is assumed that you will be able to have an impact on the ethical culture of your company. This may involve creating an ethics committee (Moon, 2019) and perhaps even serving as chair of that committee. Other activities to promote an ethical culture include systematically praising and bringing attention to ethical behavior, routinely meeting to discuss ethics issues, having guest speakers who can talk about ethics issues, and "creating contingencies that reinforce honest and principled behavior within the workplace" (Bailey & Burch, 2016, p. 168).

SENIOR BEHAVIOR ANALYST

As a seasoned behavior analyst with seniority in your company, you should be able to institute corporate policies that match and support the BACB Ethics Code for Behavior Analysts. This might be similar to the Ethics, Integrity, and Professionalism Standards now required by all organizations that are accredited by the Behavioral Health Centers of Excellence (BHCOE).[3] Their 10-point standards include staff compliance with ethical requirements, disallowing of incentives to clients for recruiting other clients, requiring policies for the exchange of gifts, and avoidance of dual relationships among others.

SUMMARY

This chapter covers the topic of ethics as a professional skill that is essential if behavior analysts are to be successful in their careers. Having integrity in every aspect of their work is necessary to gain the trust of their clients and stakeholders. Ethical challenges arise almost every day and they include conditions necessary to discontinue services such as a family berating or abusing their therapists, parents unwilling to follow through with a treatment plan, or the home environment being unsuitable for treatment. Unethical conduct by nonbehavioral colleagues presents another ethical challenge since we occasionally realize that nonbehavioral colleagues do not always adhere to our standards of treatment.

NOTES

1 www.kennedykrieger.org Internationally recognized behavioral treatment center in Baltimore.

2 Behavior Analyst Certification Board (2020). Ethics Code for Behavior Analysts. www.bacb.com/wp-content/uploads/2020/11/Ethics-Code-for-Behavior-Analysts-210902.pdf

3 https://bhcoe.org/2021/01/webinar-recap-bhcoe-ethics-integrity-professional-standards/

REFERENCES

Bailey, J. S., & Burch, M. R. (2016). *Ethics for behavior analysts* (3rd ed.). New York: Routledge, Inc.

Bailey, J. S., & Burch, M. R. (2018). *Research methods in applied behavior analysis* (2nd ed.). New York: Routledge, Inc.

Bailey, J. S., & Burch, M. R. (2022). *Ethics for behavior analysts* (4th ed.). New York: Routledge, Inc.

Behavior Analyst Certification Board. (2020). *Ethics code for behavior analysts.* Retrieved from https://bacb.com/wp-content/ethics-code-for-behavior-analysts/

Moon, M. (2019). Institutional ethics committees. *Pediatrics, 143*(5), e20190659.

4

Total Competence in Applied Behavior Analysis and in Your Specialty

I am, as I've said, merely competent. But in an age of incompetence, that makes me extraordinary.

—Billy Joel

Behavior analysis offers us a set of basic principles that explain a wide range of behavior. Our field is sufficiently robust in that it offers treatments for the complete spectrum of clients, from infants to seniors, from individuals with severe and profound disabilities to world-class athletes and Fortune 500 CEOs. The *Journal of Applied Behavior Analysis* (JABA) has provided us with more than 50 years of well-controlled studies that point to a precise methodology for measurement, a complete system for functional analysis, and a replicable and reliable treatment protocol that fulfils B. F. Skinner's dream of a validated science of behavior that can be put into service for the benefit of mankind. This strong, scientific foundation obviously puts us in an ideal position to make a significant contribution to society. The downside is that in some circumstances, we might raise the expectations of our consumers and not be able to meet them. This is not because we don't have the technology, but because our personnel are not sufficiently versed in the details for each

DOI: 10.4324/9781003265573-5

population. In short, problems arise when behavior analysts are not totally competent in an area for which they are asked to provide treatment. A behavior analyst who specialized in autism treatment in graduate school may not know exactly how to work with patients with Alzheimer's, and someone who got her practicum training in an elementary school classroom may not know how to treat a teenager with developmental disabilities who is presenting serious self-injurious behavior. Our BACB Ethics Code makes it clear that behavior analysts should not practice outside their scope of competence (BACB Code 1.05), but this doesn't prevent administrators, supervisors, parents, or others from asking for help with such cases (Bailey & Burch, 2022). The caring and compassionate behavior analyst might have a hard time turning away such requests, especially if there do not appear to be any other qualified individuals nearby.

> Blood was streaming out of Tim's ear and down the side of his cheek. It was then I realized I was in over my head.
>
> —Anonymous, a new BCBA

FRESH OUT OF GRAD SCHOOL, FIRST JOB

Our new behavior analyst (anonymous in the sidebar above) put himself in a liability situation where, under some circumstances, his professional career could have come to a screeching halt. Having *total competence in your specialty* means understanding the complexities of behavior in your area of expertise. This includes knowing what to look for in a client folder, including the medical section and understanding enough of the medical terminology to determine the severity of the condition. Grasping the technical difference between *lacerations*, *abrasions*, and *contusions*, for example, and having the professional background to inquire about the client's most recent behavioral incidents, as well as the conditions under which the injuries occurred, indicate that you are fully aware of what you are getting into when you take a case. This level of competence is needed not only for self-preservation but also to ensure the best interest of your client. If a client is injured on your watch, you must take some responsibility. If it turns out that you really were not qualified to handle the case, this could come back to haunt you.

YOUNG PROFESSIONAL (3–5 YEARS)

Having made it through your first year as a BCBA is a major accomplishment since it means that you have the basic behavioral skills necessary to cope with the routine challenges presented by clients and supervisees. However, this is no time to rest on your laurels. Instead, you should be looking ahead to develop *total* competence in the basics as you develop one or more specialties in behavior analysis.

Total Competence in Applied Behavior Analysis

To be totally competent in applied behavior analysis means that you have gone beyond the minimal requirements to pass the Behavior Analyst Certification Board (BACB) exam—way beyond. It is widely acknowledged that the exam is a test of *minimal* competence to practice in the field. Passing the BACB exam, however, does not mean that you are qualified to take on just *any* case that comes along. The expectation of leaders in the field is that you will continue to read on your own and participate in continuing education if you are a member of this proud new profession.

Expanding your knowledge of behavior analysis means keeping up with recently published books that are coming out each year, going to the annual Association for Behavior Analysis International (ABAI) conference, and attending sessions both in your specialty and in broader scope areas. ABAI has initiated the B. F. Skinner Lecture Series in which scholars and researchers indirectly related to behavior analysis are invited to present their latest data and their innovative theories related to behavior. For example, at a recent conference, you could have attended sessions titled "Treating Depression to Reduce Behavioral Risk Factors for Cardiovascular Disease: A Preventive Behavioral Medicine Perspective," "Intelligent Behaviour of Animals and Plants," and "Cannabis Dose-Effects Across Routes of Administration: Subjective, Performance, and Pharmacokinetic Differences."[1]

Each of these sessions was a mind-expanding, enriching experience where behavior analysts in attendance were challenged to formulate a worldview of behavior analysis that is intriguing, complex, and brimming with possibilities. To think that our perspective on behavior is taken seriously by behavioral scientists of all types is gratifying, and to begin to understand how everything fits together is challenging, to say the least. Attending conferences and attending sessions will bring your competence to a new level.

Monitoring Your Own Practice

In addition to keeping up with your reading and going to conferences, the next most important way that you can remain totally competent is to carefully monitor your own practice. You must collect data all the way from baseline to follow-up so you can determine if your behavior program is effective. This is a unique requirement of our field (BACB Ethics Code 2.17) that clearly separates us from the rest of the human services, and we want to make sure that we fulfill it with integrity. Seeking colleagues who will review your data is another important aspect of competence. This falls into the category of peer review. It is one thing to look at your own data and pronounce it "solid," and it is another matter to show it to an independent professional for an opinion. If you have an organized peer review committee in your area, you can use its members' oversight and feedback to maintain your skills. Peer review by other competent behavior analysts will ensure that you stay on the cutting edge of our field. You may even be able to raise the bar for your colleagues by educating them about some new techniques you learned at a conference or read about in the latest issues of *JABA* or *Behavior Analysis in Practice*.

> "What they are looking for is someone who learns quickly and who can communicate with workers who wear safety glasses, steel-toed boots, and hard hats. Can you do that?"

Developing Competence in a Specialty

In a case related to competence in performance management (PM), a brand-new master's-level behavior analyst with some basic experience in PM had an opportunity to interview for a job involving safety in the open-pit mining and steel industry. The posting was in another country, and the graduate sought advice from her major professor. "I don't know anything about mining or steel production, but I've always wanted to travel, and this job is perfect for me," she said excitedly. After reviewing the job description, the major professor asked, "What they are looking for is someone who learns quickly and who can communicate with workers who wear safety glasses, steel-toed boots, and hard hats. Can you do that?" "Absolutely," was the response. "Okay, then take the interview, and emphasize that you are a quick study and that you love meeting people. Talk about the experience you've had in a variety of business situations. And don't forget to mention that you prepared for 6 months to compete in a fundraising marathon, finished in the top 100 runners, and raised over $3,000 for charity. Finally, don't forget to ask questions about how you will be trained and the nature of your supervision."

The new graduate landed her dream job. Even though she was not competent in the open-pit mining industry, she felt comfortable with accepting the job because her consulting firm made it clear before she started that she would receive extensive training and supervision. In six months, she was fully responsible for two industrial clients and was ready to train another new consultant with her consulting firm. She reported, "They gave me two four-inch binders of information and told me I had to be fluent on the material in a week. I was able to demonstrate that I'm a quick study, and my graduate school training really paid off in this situation."

Total Competence in Your Specialty

Within applied behavior analysis, there are many specialty areas. Starting with autism and moving on to the work that is done in zoos, we can accurately say that behavior analysis specialties range from A to Z. Specialty areas within behavior analysis include but are not limited to areas as diverse as addiction, severe aggression, animal behavior, autism, behavioral gerontology, medicine, and pediatrics. Additional specialty areas include behavioral safety, clinical and developmental behavior analysis, developmental disabilities, direct instruction, elopement, gambling, health, sports issues, organizational behavior management, parent training, performance management, pica, severe destructive behavior, sex therapy, SIB (self-injurious behavior), sleep disorders, and verbal behavior.

Total competence within a specialty means that you have first defined your area of expertise as it relates to the course work you've taken, and the practicum experience you've had. Total competence also requires that you complete the necessary continuing education hours and read additional materials that will help you keep up with your specialty. If you want to be competent within a specialty area, you'll probably need to subscribe to two or three topical journals in addition to your ongoing general reading. Finally, to develop *total competence*, you will need years of experience working in the field under a range of circumstances from well-controlled clinic settings to open community placements. Here is a partial list of some of the major journals which publish single-case design studies or research specifically on behavioral disorders (Bailey & Burch, 2018, p. 39):

- *American Journal of Mental Deficiency*
- *Analysis of Verbal Behavior*
- *Behavior Analysis in Practice*
- *Behavior Change*
- *Behavior Modification*
- *Behavior Research and Therapy*
- *Behavior Therapy*
- *Behavioral Assessment*
- *Behavioral Interventions*
- *Child & Family Behavior Therapy*

- *Cognitive Therapy and Research*
- *Education and Treatment of Children*
- *Journal of Autism & Developmental Disabilities*
- *Journal of Behavior Therapy and Experimental Psychiatry*
- *Journal of Behavioral Education*
- *Journal of Organizational Behavior Management*
- *Journal of Positive Behavior Interventions*
- *Research in Autism Spectrum Disorders*

Three other journals occasionally publish behavioral studies:

- *Environment and Behavior*
- *Journal of Experimental Child Psychology*
- *Psychological Record*

Within your specialty area, as you gain years of experience, you will be able to determine which cases you can safely take and those that you need to refer to another professional. The following list can be used to determine if you are totally competent in your area of expertise:

- I was personally trained in this specialty by a Board Certified Behavior Analyst who is a recognized expert on the topic.
- I have read the most recent peer-reviewed research in the best journals on this specialized topic.
- I own the reference and textbooks considered to be the landmark works on this topic, and I have read them thoroughly.
- I have attended workshops on this specific topic in the past year.
- I can identify the experts on this topic, and I have interacted with them on more than one occasion. I can reach out to them by Zoom, phone or email if necessary.
- Colleagues regularly consult with me on their cases involving my specialty.
- I have given presentations on this topic at state or national meetings of behavior analysts.

It is in this period that many behavior analysts, now sure that this is what they want to devote their life to, consider taking time off to earn their doctorate degree and perhaps move into academia. A PhD program requires three to five years of concentrated effort, but it can be a sure way to consolidate your focus on a particular domain and contribute to the peer-reviewed literature.

MID-CAREER (6–10 YEARS)

When you reach this point in your career as a behavior analyst, it is expected that you are spending several hours each week in personal professional development keeping up with the current research in *JABA* as well as the other journals in your specialty area. You will be planning your annual calendar of the larger state and national conferences where you will be attending workshops in your specialty area. It could be that you are giving Invited Addresses and even the occasional Keynote Address. It is important at this stage for you to meet individually with your colleagues and to participate in special interest groups to remain current on the latest developments in research and practice. In some cases, you may schedule regular Zoom meetings with a distant colleague or plan a trip to visit their lab or clinic to learn about new techniques they have developed.

SENIOR BEHAVIOR ANALYST

As a senior behavior analyst, it is expected that you will be at the top of your game. While there are Senior Behavior Analysts who choose to have a career providing treatment to clients, be aware that for the Senior Behavior Analyst, the sky is the limit. As a Senior Behavior Analyst, you are likely to be a recognized expert in two or more specialties who is sought after for advice on clinical matters as well as consulting on corporate organizational concerns.

SUMMARY

This chapter covers the stages of expected competency from straight out of graduate school to senior behavior analyst status. We describe the competencies that one achieves initially such as working directly with clients while providing therapy and then moving up to providing supervision to those who do hands-on work with clients. One lesson learned is that there is a scope of competence to be respected and when you are given a case that is beyond that scope, the most ethical action is to return-to-sender with a note as to the rationale. When you reach the point of having one to two years working as a full-time BCBA, there is an expectation that you will have total competence in the basic procedures with a standard general population of clients. With two years or more of experience as a BCBA, you might be expected to develop expertise in a specialty area by going to conferences, enrolling in workshops, and working with a mentor.

NOTE

1 (43rd Annual Convention Association for Behavior Analysis International, Denver, 2017. www.abainternational.org/events/program-details/search-result.aspx?intConvId=48&by=BFSkinner)

FOR FURTHER READING

Behavior Analysis in Practice. Kalamazoo, MI: Association for Behavior Analysis International.

Behavior Analyst Certification Board. (2020). *Ethics code for behavior analysts.* Retrieved from https://bacb.com/wp-content/ethics-code-for-behavior-analysts/

Behavioral Interventions. New York: John Wiley & Sons.

Journal of Applied Behavior Analysis. Bloomington, IN: Society for the Experimental Analysis of Behavior.

Journal of Organizational Behavior Management. Philadelphia, PA: Taylor & Francis Group.

Skinner, B. F. (1953). *Science and human behavior.* New York: Macmillan.

REFERENCES

Bailey, J. S., & Burch, M. R. (2018). *Research methods in applied behavior analysis* (2nd ed.). New York: Routledge, Inc.

Bailey, J. S., & Burch, M. R. (2022). *Ethics for behavior analysts* (4th ed.). New York: Routledge, Inc.

5

"Think Function"

What is lacking is a satisfactory "causal" or functional treatment.

—B. F. Skinner

My sickness is that I'm fascinated by human behavior, by what's underneath the surface, by the worlds inside people.

—Johnny Depp

FRESH OUT OF GRAD SCHOOL, FIRST JOB

"Think Function"[1] is a maxim that reminds us that every behavior problem has a solution and that finding one starts with understanding the *motivation* for a behavior. In lay terms, there is a *cause* for what people do (Skinner, 1957, p. 5) and if we can find the cause we might be able to develop a treatment or intervention to change the behavior. In our world, the cause we are

"Think Function" is a maxim that reminds us that every behavior problem has a solution and that finding one starts with understanding the *motivation* for a behavior.

DOI: 10.4324/9781003265573-6

looking for is usually proximal and hiding somewhere in the environment. A child who whines is doing so because it gets them what they want ("Cocoa Puffs, I want Cocoa Puffs"), or gets them out of something they hate doing ("I don't want to go to bed . . ."). Average citizens are not trained to see these variables and they often resort to labeling ("He's just a whiny kid; he's always been that way . . .") or blaming ("She's lazy just like her dad; it's all his fault, he's a bad role model . . ."). Behavior analysts are famous for making this discovery, and we tend to apply it to both our clinical cases and larger organizational issues that can be looked at through this lens. This chapter describes some of the non-clinical applications where behavior analysts encounter "Think Function" throughout their careers.

One of the first evidence-based lessons of grad school is that doing a functional analysis (FA) (Iwata, Dorsey, Slifer, Bauman, & Richman, 1982, 1994) is essential to the development of a behavior plan. As a student, conducting one or more of these sophisticated assessments is part of your preparation for your career in behavior analysis. This can produce a rather myopic view of behavior where there is a focus on a specific behavior that a client is exhibiting and the immediate contingencies in the environment (escape, attention, etc.) that seem to produce it. This is a natural and appropriate reaction in a clinical or educational setting, and it feels good to be operating as a behavioral *scientist.* Having conducted a few functional analyses during your supervised placement allows you to understand the power of the multi-element design and appreciate even more the multitude of FA studies being published in nearly every issue of *JABA*. Learning to read graphs showing differentiation and discern which variables are truly relevant can be an amazing accomplishment and should lead to interventions that work quickly with amazing results.

Functional Analysis of Stakeholder Behavior

It is only when you move to phase two and try to see the results of your FA that reality sets in. If it was only you implementing the behavior plan, there would be no problem. However, it turns out that RBTs, parents, teachers, and other stakeholders are responsible for this stage. This is where the true meaning of "Think Function" sets in (This motto in logo format created by the first author for the Florida Association for Behavior Analysis is shown in Figure 5.1). You must find out where the breakdown was: was your training not thorough? Was the task too difficult? Is there some response cost involved in executing the behavior plan? Are you not providing enough feedback and reinforcement? All of these are possibilities, and you need to find out which one is relevant if your plan is going to be a success. When it comes to evaluating your expertise in training caregivers, you will probably have to rely on your own direct observations and related data. If others fail to carry out your behavior plan as designed, nothing can take the place of you directly observing the implementation of the program. If you are not using BST (Behavior Skills Training), don't be surprised if *they just don't get it*. They may be missing some steps that are critical to the plan, and if doesn't work for them, they quit. Or there may be too many steps, or you did not present them in a logical order. You will be able to find where things went wrong by conducting direct observations, so this is your first strategy. Under normal circumstances, you will have demonstrated the behavior plan to the RBTs or caregivers and then gradually faded out and

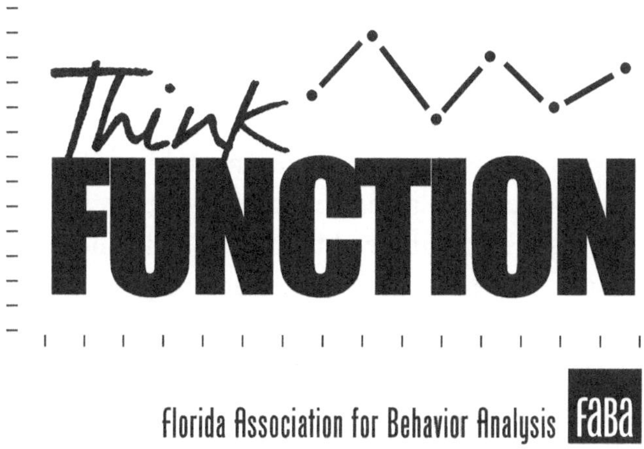

Figure 5.1 Graphic of the FABA "Think Function" slogan.

handed it off to them. If you faded too quickly, this could also be a problem. One "function" that is most troublesome is their failure to *buy in* to the whole concept of behavior change. This should not be a problem with RBTs but could be with parents or teachers. If you moved too quickly from your assessment of the problem behavior to your proposed behavior plan without answering their questions and listening to their input, this form of dissent might have been overlooked. If this is the case, you basically need to back up and try again. Consider modifying the program and its training and then try to be persuasive about the importance of the endeavor and their key role in the solution. Often resistance to new ideas can be overcome by a good clear demonstration of how your suggestion works, especially if there is an obvious effect. The resistance of those who are assigned to implement behavior plans has a function. Find the function and make the necessary modifications, and you should be on your way.

Functional Analysis of Supervisee Behavior

Another population you will encounter in your first job that may present behavior challenges is your group of supervisees. As a new BCBA supervisor, this may come as something of a shock, especially if you were once a great supervisee who had a top-notch supervisor who trained you well. But you may be presented with RBTs and trainees who do not appear to be well trained, highly motivated, or entirely professional. Rather than blaming them for their shortcomings, "Think Function." This could be a prompt for you to consider that their preparation to be an RBT may have been lax and incomplete. This will mean that your "supervisor" job will need to expand to include re-training and remediation. Simply giving feedback may not be enough to compensate for a slacker attitude. Instruction, modeling, role-play, practice, AND feedback will probably be necessary to bring them up to your standard. A lack of motivation points to the absence of sufficient reinforcement to sustain the difficult task of working with clients, hour after hour, day after day for relatively low wages. While you may not be able to do much about wages in your new position, over time as you move up in the organization, you might be able to make a difference in this area.

> Say to yourself, "I need to Think Function."

Functional Analysis of Your Own Behavior

Think Function applies everywhere from parents being late in dropping off their child at the clinic (car broke down, someone overslept), to breaking local news stories (a five-car pile-up on I-10), to international relations (peace talks have failed in Geneva). It also comes into play for your own behavior (What happened to that New Year's resolution to give up smoking?) as well as your clients, their parents, your colleagues, supervisors, and college instructors. What if your supervisor has a habit of forgetting to bring the EVF (Experience Verification Form) to your supervision sessions or forgets the meeting altogether; the bookkeeper routinely loses the paperwork you turn in, and your RBT's data collection is incomplete? On and on it goes. These are all behaviors to worry about and complain about, but in addition to that if you are going to correct the situation you need to know the controlling variables. Say to yourself, "I need to *Think Function*." You could ask for a meeting with your supervisor or have a talk with the bookkeeper, but nothing is going to change unless you understand the controlling variable(s) and begin the process of changing the environment systematically to produce a different outcome.

As you move up from trainee to becoming a full-fledged BCBA, and then possibly to a BCBA Supervisor, you need to be prepared to conduct informal functional analyses of your own professional behavior as well as the behavior of people with whom you work. This will not look like the traditional experimental functional analysis of course, but the purpose is the same. Before we had the *Iwata Model* of functional analysis, there was the *Trial and Error Method* of finding controlling variables. This will be your most likely tactic and combined with the *Least Restrictive Method*, this should get you started. While still in grad school, a great place to start understanding the search for functional variables is with your own behavior and we recommend beginning with your personal and professional habits. Find a close friend or student colleague who will be truthful with you. Ask that person what you can improve in terms of dress, grooming, and presentation skills with clients and stakeholders as well as supervisors. Most of the time, your professors are unlikely to give this type of feedback. Be prepared for some frank discussions about your appearance (e.g., too much aftershave, excessive perfume, not enough deodorant) and your demeanor with clients, parents, and stakeholders. Your supervisor will presumably take care of your handling of client behaviors.

YOUNG PROFESSIONAL (3–5 YEARS)

After you have been on the job for a year or two, the stakes are somewhat higher for your "*Think Function*" repertoire. If you have followed the guidelines suggested earlier, you should now have a robust history of reinforcement for looking for the functions of behavior and misbehavior in other people. Hopefully, you will have overcome all your own significant flaws, faults, and foibles, and you should have learned effective ways of persuading your clients to participate in the behavior change enterprise actively and happily. By now, you should have many accomplishments under your belt, and perhaps even a reputation as a successful behavior analyst. As a young professional, your next task is to look around your organization and determine where there are glitches in the service-delivery system. By this point in your career, you should have adopted the "Think Function" motto and made it part of your daily interactions with clients, caregivers, and those that you supervise, as well as colleagues at work.

MID-CAREER (6–10 YEARS)

At mid-career, you will have managed hundreds of clinical cases and just as many RBTs and other supervisees. Your "Think

Function" repertoire may work almost automatically now. When you hear parents describe the behavior of their child, you will immediately reflect on similar cases you have handled and be able to predict a pattern. Your extensive experience may also have engendered a certain amount of skepticism and your need to observe the child or adolescent yourself becomes a priority. Through direct observation, it may be possible to "see" the function operating, which allows you to direct your team to find ways of working therapeutically with the client.

SENIOR BEHAVIOR ANALYST

As a senior behavior analyst with more than a decade of experience, you should have a full appreciation of the impact that behavior analysis can have not only on children and their families but also on the potential for an even greater impact on your community. With your experience and connections and an awareness of issues in your community, it is possible that you can think about larger concerns such as homelessness, unemployment, drugs, education, voter registration, crime, and more. Each of these can be approached from the "Think Function" vantage point, and you may want your organization to become involved in a citizen task force that will attempt to address not just short-term solutions but underlying factors that can be rectified by a better understanding of the contingencies that have generated them in the first place. Dr. Bill Heward's behavioral initiative on climate change and sustainable practices is a good model for senior behavior analysts who want to make a difference (Heward & Chance, 2010).

SUMMARY

This chapter introduces the concept of functional analysis. Functional analysis (FA) is a way of discovering the motivation for any behavior under consideration and it provides one way for the new BCBA to use this maxim to work with their clients' families and stakeholders. For young professionals, there are usually higher expectations by their agencies for a greater level of involvement with certain broader issues such as recruitment and retention of quality RBTs, improving training techniques, and dealing with ethical issues arising from interactions with clients. Once you have been in the field for half-a-dozen years or so, there is an expectation that you will be able to easily understand the motivations of client families and stakeholders and overcome obstacles that lead to their full cooperation.

NOTE

1 This motto created by the first author for the 1987 FABA Conference where Dr. Brian Iwata was the Keynote Speaker.

FOR FURTHER READING

Charlton, S. R., Detrich, R., Dixon, M. R., Magoon, M. A., & Critchfield, T. S. (2013). Getting the public to accept behavior analysis as a route to sustainability. *Inside Behavior Analysis*, *5*(1), 15–16.

Geller, E. S. (2013). Actively caring for the environment: How applied behavior analysis can do more for sustainability. *Inside Behavior Analysis*, *5*(1), 11–12.

Heward, W. L., & Chance, P. (Guest Eds.). (2010). Special section: The human response to climate change: Ideas from behavior analysis. *The Behavior Analyst*, *33*, 145–206.

Kareiva, P. (2012). Resurrecting the environmental movement. *Invited address at behavior change for a sustainable world conference.* Columbus, OH: Association for Behavior Analysis International.

Knott, S., Kernan, D., Luke, M., & Alavosius, M. (2012). Distributing green practices: Sustainability in a supply chain. *Paper presented at the 38th annual meeting of the association for behavior analysis international.* Seattle, WA.

Komiyama, H., & Takeuchi, K. (2006). Sustainability science: Building a new discipline. *Sustainability Science*, *1*, 1–6.

Lattal, D. (2013). Time to recognize green behavior standards for corporations? *Inside Behavior Analysis*, *5*(1), 14–15.

Luke, M., Alavosius, M. P., Newsome, W. D., & Leeming, E. M. (2011). Climate change and human behavior: An undergraduate/graduate course in environmental psychology at University of Nevada, Reno. *Paper presented at the 37th annual meeting of the association for behavior analysis international.* Denver, CO.

Mingle, J. (2012). Scientists ask blunt question on everyone's mind. *Slate*. Retrieved December 12, 2012, from www.slate.com/articles/health_and_science/science/2012/12/is_earth_f_ked_at_2012_agu_meeting_ scientists_consider_advocacy_activism.single.html#pagebreak_anchor_2

Provenza, P. (2013). Connecting humans, animals and landscapes for the good of all. *Inside Behavior Analysis*, *5*(1), 13–14.

Scherer, G. (2012). Climate science predictions prove too conservative. *Scientific American*. Retrieved December 12, 2012, from www.scientificamerican.com/article.cfm?id=climate-science-predictions-prove-too-conservative

Sidman, M. (2007). The analysis of behavior: What's in it for us? *Journal of the Experimental Analysis of Behavior*, *39*, 309–315.

Stratton, J. P. (2013). Building bridges across disciplines to support sustainable practices: The role of behavior analysis. *Inside Behavior Analysis*, *5*(1), 17–18.

Thompson, L. G. (2010). Climate change: The evidence and our options. *The Behavior Analyst*, *33*, 153–170.

Thompson, L. G. (2013). The greatest challenge of global climate change: An inconvenient truth meets the inconvenienced mind. *Inside Behavior Analysis*, *5*(1), 8–9.

Wilhite, C. (2012). Three more projects from Fresno State. *Paper presented at the 38th annual meeting of the association for behavior analysis international*. Seattle, WA.

REFERENCES

Heward, W. L., & Chance, P. (2010). Introduction: Dealing with what is. *Behavior Analyst*, *33*, 145–151. https://doi.org/10.1007/BF03392210

Iwata, B. A., Dorsey, M. F., Slifer, K. J., Bauman, K. E., & Richman, G. S. (1982). Toward a functional analysis of self-injury. *Analysis and Intervention in Developmental Disabilities*, *2*, 3–20. https://doi.org/10.1016/0270-4684(82)90003-9

Iwata, B. A., Dorsey, M. F., Slifer, K. J., Bauman, K. E., & Richman, G. S. (1994). Toward a functional analysis of self-injury. *Journal of Applied Behavior Analysis*, *27*, 197–209. http://doi.org/10.1901/jaba.1994.27-197

Skinner, B. F. (1957). *Verbal behavior*. Englewood Cliffs, NJ: Prentice Hall.

Unit

Two

The Basic Behavioral Repertoire

At a workshop for ABA supervisors, a BCBA-D talked about some of her supervisees who were BCBAs with one to two years of experience:

> They are learning the structure necessary to supervise RBTs. Even though they are BCBAs, some only have a year or two of experience, so I still need to monitor them to see that they are checking that the protocol of the behavior plan is followed. And I need to make sure they are taking data and comparing it to the RBTs' data—this is a must. We believe that providing feedback and training is helping our BCBAs develop leadership skills.
>
> We work with a diverse group of clients. Some of our BCBAs came to us from smaller cities where there isn't much diversity. When working in client homes, we expect all staff to be culturally

DOI: 10.4324/9781003265573-7

responsive—they need to learn about and be sensitive to the cultures of everyone.

Above all, our BCBAs need to be strong advocates for clients and their families. We accept nothing less.

6

Deliberate, Ethical Supervision

This is awful. Do it again.
—Henry A. Kissinger

FRESH OUT OF GRAD SCHOOL, FIRST JOB

Each grad school experience is unique for every BCBA who completes a master's program. Some will have had a supervisor who took an interest in them, developed a personal relationship, and fostered their career (LeBlanc, Sellers, & Ala'i, 2020, pp. 3–65). Others had a supervisor with poor interpersonal skills who observed them irregularly and did not provide effective feedback. Others may have had a spurious supervision experience that consisted primarily of a "How are you doing?" in the hallway or on the phone followed by, "Drop your forms off and I'll sign them for you." Unfortunately, the supervision experience in the formative years of a graduate program will likely predict the practices of the new BCBA. For this reason, in this chapter we will describe what we believe are the *minimum standards of practice* that every new BCBA should employ regardless of their own personal training experience. We assume that by this time, you have met the experience standards set by the BACB (Supervisor Training Curriculum Outline (2.0, 2018b), BACB Handbook, 2022).

DOI: 10.4324/9781003265573-8

We believe it is useful to conceptualize supervision from the bottom up rather than top-down, i.e., first, what is the *primary* purpose of supervision? In a word, it is *Quality*. The most important purpose of supervision is to ensure that the client is receiving the precise behavior plan that was envisioned by the BCBA supervisor and delivered by the RBT or trainee. High-quality supervision can only be achieved by close-up, in-person, consistent monitoring and shaping of the RBT or trainee's performance to assure that the standards are high, and the expected outcomes achieved.

According to the RBT Task List (BACB, 2018a, 2nd ed.) there are six types of tasks that are required (BACB, 2018a, 2nd ed., p. 1): 1) *Measurement* 2) *Assessment*, 3) *Skill Acquisition*, 4) *Behavior Reduction*, 5) *Documentation and Reporting*, and 6) *Professional Conduct and Scope of Practice*, i.e., with regard to training, RBTs are required to collect data for each session and enter the data in graphic form. The RBT is to be supervised in such a way that these six tasks are carried out reliably, and with integrity, so the client receives the full benefit of the behavioral services to which they are entitled. Treatment integrity and accountability are required by the funding agencies to justify payment.

Supervision must result in a measurable outcome of the highest quality for the client with a specified value to the payer

Viewed in this way, basic supervision is not a task that allows for much variability in the manner of implementation. Supervision must result in a measurable outcome of the highest quality for the client with a specified value to the payer. The RBT must implement the acquisition or reduction program with measured integrity and high inter-observer agreement (IOA) with their BCBA supervisor. Next, they must accurately measure the client's response to the behavior-change intervention on a per-session basis. Measuring the client's response to the implementation can be considered a permanent product. Measurement is critical in this analysis since data is fed upward to the BCBA and the organization as a measure of the appropriateness of the plan, the effectiveness of the RBT, and the supervisor. If the data is inaccurate, it can lead to changes in the intervention that are unnecessary or possibly have deeper implications, e.g., if the behavior plan is "not working" then medications may be prescribed, restraints may be employed, or the client discharged.

The most important purpose of supervision is to ensure that the client is receiving the precise behavior plan that was envisioned by the BCBA supervisor and delivered by the RBT or trainee.

Supervision Basics

Supervision consists of four required tasks: 1) observe the RBT and take data to determine if they are following the training protocol, 2) observe the RBT and take data to determine if they are implementing the behavior-change program properly, 3) determine if the supervisor's measures match that of the RBT or trainee, and 4) provide the necessary feedback and training. As a side note, we

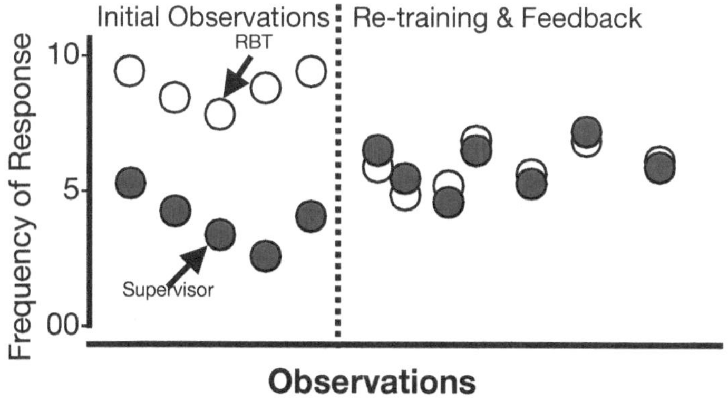

Figure 6.1 This figure shows the tasks for which the RBT is responsible and how the BCBA Supervisor determines if the behavior-change protocol has been implemented with integrity, and if the RBT's measurement of the client's behavior matches their count.

certainly do not recommend following the feedback style of Dr. Kissinger that was mentioned previously.

If there is a disparity in step 3, then re-training and feedback is in order as shown in Figures 6.2 and 6.3. This process can and should be used to evaluate the supervisor's effectiveness (Garza, McGee, Schenk, & Wiskirchen, 2018).

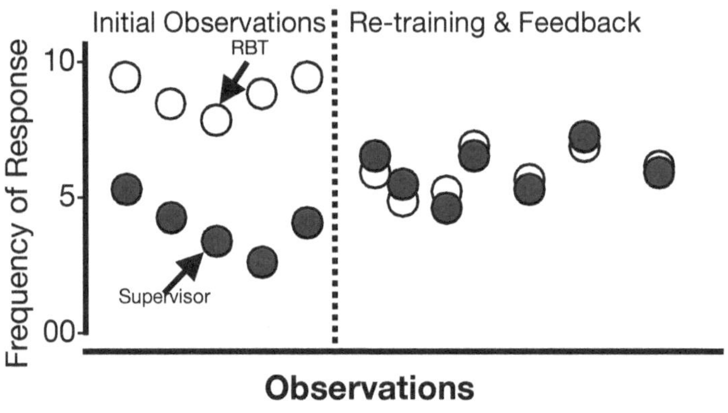

Figure 6.2 This figure shows how the RBT's count of their client's behavior differed greatly from that of the supervisor during the initial observations. After re-training and feedback, the RBT's count closely matched the supervisors and acceptable IOA of client behavior was achieved.

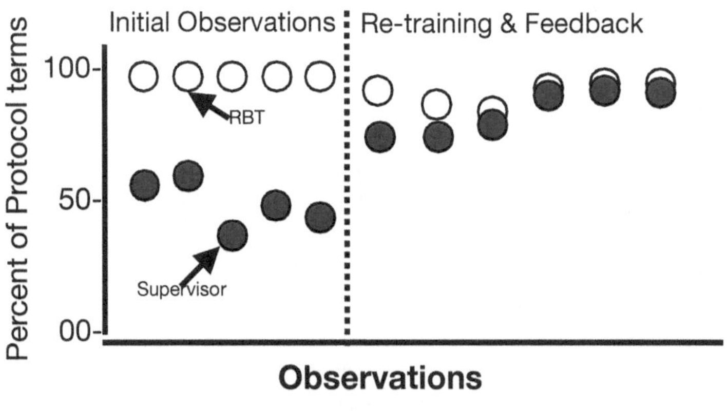

Figure 6.3 This figure shows the RBT's self-estimate of their treatment integrity at very nearly 100%, but the supervisor indicates that the RBT is greatly overestimating their success in following the behavior plan. After re-training and feedback, the RBT's treatment integrity improves and nearly matches that of the supervisor.

Beyond Basics

As described in detail in LeBlanc et al. (2020), once the RBTs and supervisees have reached criterion and have demonstrated maintenance of the protocol following accurate behavior measurement and graphing, it will be time to begin expanding their repertoires. At this point, supervision will involve a great deal of behavior shaping (see Chapter 12). Supervisors will need to include additional professional and ethical skills as well as more advanced behavioral concepts (LeBlanc et al., 2020, pp. 4–13). They will also need to learn how to think like a behavior analyst (Bailey & Burch, 2022). Thinking like a behavior analyst involves conceptualizing and contextualizing behavior problems and their solutions, developing interpersonal, problem-solving, and troubleshooting skills, and learning where to seek help when it is needed. The BACB has spelled out the essential steps of training a supervisor (Behavior Analyst Certification Board, 2018b). These include being "able to state the purpose of supervision to the supervisee or trainee," describe the outcomes of "ineffective supervision," "prepare for the supervisory relationship," "have a plan for supervision content and evaluation of competence," and be able to "create a positive relationship" with the RBT, trainee, or supervisee. In addition, a supervisor needs to know how to use behavioral skills training (BST) in their training, evaluate the effects of that training (including directly observing their trainee and evaluating the fidelity of interventions as described previously in supervision basics), assess their professionalism, and discuss ethics. These are the general categories of skills that the new supervisor needs to acquire. When the sub-items are included, there are more than 200 items that are contained in the training curriculum for supervisors. These skills have been broken down into small steps in a comprehensive checklist format for ease of access for the new supervisor and trainee (Jurgens, Cordova, & Cruz, 2021).

Ethical Supervision and the New BCBA

A quick review of the BACB Ethics Code provides the basis for the proposed term *Ethical Supervision*, which can be defined as meeting Ethics Codes 4.01–4.12 (BACB Ethics Code for Behavior Analysts, 2020b, pp. 15–16). Specifically, **Codes 4.06 Providing Supervision and Training, 4.08 Performance Monitoring and Feedback**, and **4.10 Evaluating Effects of Supervision and Training** encompass what has been described earlier as minimal requirements for ethical supervision. As a new BCBA, your first supervision assignments should focus on these important tasks with your new supervision team. If you are inheriting a team of RBTs, you will probably start with direct observations of the RBTs with their current behavior-change plans to determine if they are closely following the plan and taking accurate data on the client. This will be followed by the training necessary to bring them up to your standard.

YOUNG PROFESSIONAL (3–5 YEARS)

As you become established in your new position, you will no doubt have discovered the scheduling problems, competing responsibilities, and internal company contingencies that could impair your ability to be an effective, ethical supervisor. Your challenge will be to learn how to overcome and circumvent these trials. If you are focused on the effective implementation of the behavior-change interventions that you write, the outcome should be steady progress on the part of your clients as well as professional growth by your RBTs and trainees. Most programs will have monthly Case Management Reviews where you can bring up client cases to showcase effective interventions as well as discuss problems that have come up in the process. This will be an opportunity to share your method of supervision that has produced these results and hopefully spread the word about ethical supervision.

MID-CAREER (6–10 YEARS)

When you have passed the 5-year mark at your organization, your reputation as an experienced and successful supervisor may have elevated you to a new position as Consulting

Supervisor (BACB, 2021) or possibly Director of Training. In this capacity, you will be in a position to guide the new BCBAs toward the ethical supervision model. In addition, you may have developed systems for collecting RBT data on client behavior change that will accurately represent their progress to funding agencies.

SENIOR BEHAVIOR ANALYST

With a full decade behind you, it is likely that you will be in a management position where you will have some influence with the CEO (or *be* the CEO) or COO and board of directors who make policy decisions and allocate funds for program expansion. If this is the case, you will be able to take your years of experience in training new BCBA supervisors to develop new training strategies that emphasize the basics and expand beyond all of the other areas of importance to supervisors.

SUMMARY

This chapter covers the very essential skill of supervision. Supervision is a skill that all practicing behavior analysts who are BCBAs must master if they are going to be effective on their first jobs. The range of behaviors required to be effective is quite large, but the basics must be mastered first. Since the RBT or trainee is the primary person responsible for the delivery of services, there is an obligation to make sure that this task is completed ethically with fluency, competence, and effectiveness. This standard can only be met through direct observation and simultaneous data collection of the RBT working with the client. Once the data is collected, training to correct any deficiencies is implemented to guarantee that the client is receiving the services promised to the funding agencies. Only when your RBTs or trainees are following the protocols and accurately reporting the results of their training is it time to move on to more advanced aspects of supervision. Advancing ethical supervision practices can become more widespread once a BCBA moves up in the ranks of the organization.

REFERENCES

Bailey, J. S., & Burch, M. R. (2022). *How to think like a behavior analyst* (2nd ed.). New York: Routledge, Inc.

Behavior Analyst Certification Board. (2018a). *RBT task list* (2nd ed.). Littleton, CO: Author.

Behavior Analyst Certification Board. (2018b). *Supervision training curriculum outline (2.0).* Littleton, CO: Author.

Behavior Analyst Certification Board. (2018a). *BCBA/BCaBA experience standards.* Littleton, CO: Author.

Behavior Analyst Certification Board. (2020b). *Ethics code for behavior analysts.* Littleton, CO: Author.

Behavior Analyst Certification Board. (2021). *Consulting supervisor requirements for new BCBAs supervising fieldwork.* Littleton, CO: Author.

Behavior Analyst Certification Board. (2022). *Board certified behavior analyst® handbook.* Littleton, CO: Author.

Garza, K. L., McGee, H. M., Schenk, Y. A., & Wiskirchen, R. R. (2018). Some tools for carrying out a proposed process for supervising experience hours for aspiring board certified behavior analysts®. *Behavior Analysis in Practice, 11*, 62–70. https://doi.org/10.1007/s40617-017-0186-8

Jurgens, H., Cordova, K., & Cruz, Y. (2021). *The ABA supervision handbook: A guide to quality fieldwork experience.* Ormond Beach, FL: WND Press.

LeBlanc, L. A., Sellers, T. P., & Ala'i, S. (2020). *Building and sustaining meaningful and effective relationships as a supervisor and mentor.* Cornwall on Hudson, NY: Sloan Publishing.

7
Leadership in ABA

FRESH OUT OF GRAD SCHOOL, FIRST JOB

> The single most important leadership function is to create a focus for the group's behavior.
>
> —Aubrey Daniels

In behavioral terms "leadership" entails the behavior of someone who can encourage followers to engage in productive work or another outcome such as sports or political victories. As Daniels and Daniels (2005, p. 13) have said, "The single most important leadership function is to create a focus for the group's behavior." From our perspective, becoming a leader then involves one person working with other people that have been trained, directed, and *motivated* to engage in tasks that they otherwise do not prefer. Providing the motivation to engage in the undertaking must be *the* most significant contribution of a behavioral approach. One more thing is necessary for leadership to make sense. The person who is the leader must have some idea of the behaviors that are wanted from the others. This is usually described as having a *vision* or idea of the behavior in which the leader would like to see others engage as well as the anticipated outcome. Vision is difficult to quantify or even define behaviorally, but it is certainly

DOI: 10.4324/9781003265573-9

possible to create a list of measurable behaviors that are related to the leader's vision.

> **Leadership is the process of prompting, training, and reinforcing the behavior of others so they can complete measurable tasks.**

There are usually not many opportunities to acquire leadership skills while in a graduate program in ABA since most programs justifiably stress the methodology and behavior science aspects of behavior analysis. Yet upon graduation, the new BCBA will be expected to take on some leadership responsibilities in their first full-time position. This will primarily happen in the context of on-the-job training, and it could definitely be a hit-or-miss proposition. Thousands of books have been written on *leadership*. These are mostly based on the book author's experience, their own definition of the term, and their personal theories of how leadership works. Since leadership is not a behavioral term that has been operationalized and there is no ABA research on leadership, we usually use extrapolations from other parts of the field. Probably the closest to ABA is Performance Management (PM). PM has been applying the basic principles of behavior in business and industry for over 50 years. The PM literature is heavily driven by a few basic contingencies of reinforcement. These involve training, antecedent stimuli as prompts, social and tangible feedback, plus a wide variety of consequences in an even wider array of work settings (Daniels & Bailey, 2014). Basically, leadership is the process of prompting, training, and reinforcing the behavior of others so they can complete measurable tasks.

Defining Leadership Behaviorally

Most of the literature on this topic tells us that good leaders are intelligent and enthusiastic; they have charisma, and lead by example. We're told that good leaders are not afraid to take risks, and that they know how to overcome obstacles. Emotional stability is another characteristic frequently listed for good leaders. When the going gets tough and there is a tremendous amount of frustration in the workplace, good leaders are even-keeled. They instill trust, they have integrity, and they empower the people around them. Good leaders have vision, they see the "big picture," envision a future outcome, and they know how to guide a department, a whole company, or an entire sports league. While these general characteristics certainly make for interesting reading, behavior analysts who want to develop leadership skills know that to be effective, they must translate these traits into observable behaviors. As you are working in behavior analysis, you can adopt some specific behaviors that will help you develop and eventually assume a leadership role.

On their first job out of grad school, BCBAs will be expected to *lead* supervisees and trainees through a series of tasks to meet the fieldwork requirements of the BACB. These tasks have now been operationalized which will make this process much more feasible (Jurgens, Cordova, & Cruz, 2021) but there remains the task of prompting the behavior, possibly modelling it for the trainee, and providing feedback, along with some manipulation of a MO (motivating operation) to reinforce the acquisition and routine production of the skill. In this regard, leadership looks a lot like *behavior shaping*, which is definitely a behavioral process. If one wanted to become a leader, it would be wise to start with one person to see if they could persuade that person to engage in a measurable task and if so, then expand to two people, then three, and so on. Leadership doesn't have to be a majestic and mysterious concept; it simply needs to be analyzed and operationalized like other concepts so we can make sense and good use of it.

Leadership Behaviors: How to Get Started

To prepare yourself to be a leader in your organization, you should observe the current leaders in action and determine if your values match theirs. If your values match, then you'll need to explore ways of demonstrating that you can in fact be a leader. Those who are chosen by an administration to be leaders such as a clinical director selecting BCBAs to become supervisors, clearly have the trust of those in the current leadership hierarchy. If the administrators choose you, it means that they have had a good look at your leadership repertoire and believe that you support the organization, understand its mission, and have the same values.

Acquiring leadership-related behavior shaping skills on a small scale makes supervision a great learning opportunity for early-career behavior analysts.

Supervision as Leadership

For behavior analysts who are beginning their careers, one example of leadership on a small scale involves training and supervising upcoming RBTs who are accruing their supervision hours. All of the elements of leadership are required here, but on a small and manageable scale since you will be dealing with these supervisees one-on-one. You will expect supervisees to quickly acquire and demonstrate new behavioral skills, and perhaps more importantly, you will need to provide the motivation for them to do so. As mentioned earlier, motivating people to learn new skills and actively engage in tasks that do not produce immediate reinforcers is a part of leadership that is usually omitted from the general leadership literature. Acquiring leadership/behavior shaping skills on a small scale makes supervision a great learning opportunity for early career behavior analysts. If you find that you enjoy this experience and find it rewarding to train the next generation of behavior analysts, then you are on your way.

YOUNG PROFESSIONAL (3–5 YEARS)

Successive Approximations to Leadership

Volunteering for a project that needs to be completed on a short timeline is one good way to test yourself and gain some experience. As a project leader, you'll be guiding others to complete tasks on time and in a coordinated fashion. This kind of activity on your part signals to the present leadership that you have a desire to move up in the organization. Short-term leadership experiences also allow you to learn how to quickly evaluate colleagues and other volunteers and to determine how best to use their skills. These are all good qualities of a leader.

Another characteristic of leaders that is critical to their success is integrity, a commitment to a set of values that is unwavering in the face of pressure from all sides. John Wooden coached UCLA to 10 National Collegiate Athletic Association national championships in 12 years, achieving a distinction that was unmatched in the history of basketball. When asked about his success, he described two sets of rules that his father taught him and his brothers that guided him throughout his 40-year college basketball coaching career: "Never lie; never cheat; never steal. Don't whine; don't complain; don't make excuses" (Wooden & Jamison, 2005, p. 71).

Visible Leadership: Participating in and Running a Meeting

For the behavior analyst consultant, one of the most frequent opportunities to demonstrate leadership ability will be in the numerous meetings that occur in any organization. As a new employee, you will probably be asked to attend these gatherings where you can observe how the organization runs and how the leadership conducts itself. You won't be asked to do much initially, so observing and taking notes is appropriate. Meetings can provide an opportunity for you to practice your business etiquette (see Chapter 1), show some assertiveness, (see Chapter 8) and demonstrate your newly acquired leadership skills.

One tip regarding your behavior in meetings involves understanding the protocol of timing. It is recommended that you always show up a little early; ten minutes is about right for a new employee. With this standard, you'll probably be the first person in the room and will have your choice of seating. You'll want to take a seat where you can make eye contact with the chair of the session but not sit so close as to make it appear that you are "sucking up." As people arrive, you can practice your social skills by acknowledging them. Introduce yourself if you don't know who they are; they will appreciate this gesture, and it will put other new people at ease. For example, say, "I'm Jill Harper, the new behavior analyst. I work for Jane on the ESE project that she's starting." It is appropriate for you to hand out business cards at this time. If they have cards, you can get one from each person. For people who don't have cards, be sure to write down their information (i.e., name, agency, job title, what they do, and a phone number or email address).

When the chair of the meeting arrives, take your seat, and watch what happens as she starts the meeting. Look for good leadership skills: Do people immediately cease their small talk and get down to business? Does she have to "shush" the group to quiet the room? Is there an agenda? If there is an agenda, ideally, it should have been shared via TM or email 24 hours beforehand. Watch to see if the chair specifies a time limit for the meeting; this is a good sign. Many companies want a record of what went on in the meeting, and a good chair will assign someone to take minutes.

People can be difficult to manage at meetings. They get off task, they go on too long, they are vague in their offerings or suggestions, they don't speak up, and they start bickering among themselves. The responsibility for managing all this falls on the chair. As a new employee, you can note which people present which problems. Good leaders are clear about their objectives for a meeting in terms of both the outcomes and the meeting behaviors: "I have five items for us to discuss today, and I want to be out of here in one hour, so please stay on task and help me move this along. Our first item is . . ." Some big, fast-moving companies such as Google put an image of a large ticking clock on a screen that counts down from the time allotted to keep everyone focused.

MID-CAREER (6–10 YEARS)

As a mid-career behavior analyst, as you might expect, the expectations for leadership evolve to a larger scale. At this point, you will have led several teams of RBTs and supervisees through dozens of cases and you will have encountered most of the problems dealing with clients that you will ever see. At mid-career, you may be ready to step up in your organization to a position such as a regional director or clinical director. As a regional director, you may be charged with growing the organization while expanding the vision of quality behavioral services on a larger scale. As a clinical director, you will be *leading* newer behavior analysts in possibly new directions. For example, you may be branching out to serve different client populations or working to streamline the admissions process. In this position, you will be responsible for growing the behavioral department, monitoring budgets, and reviewing the behavioral services to make sure you are meeting client needs. Leadership at this level involves recruiting new BCBAs and setting up internships with local graduate programs.

Newer problems encountered by senior behavior analysts in the C-suite include concern over cyber threats, increasing competition from corporate interests, and value-based payment or pay for performance.

SENIOR BEHAVIOR ANALYST

Many if not all senior behavior analysts will be in leadership positions by the time they have been in the field for a decade or more. Depending on the size of the organization this may mean being CEO, VP (Vice President), or a member of the BOD (Board of Directors) of the company. At this level much of the work involves personnel decisions, financial strategies, and regulatory policy (rulemaking). Newer problems encountered by senior behavior analysts in the c-suite include concern over cyber threats, increasing competition from corporate interests, and value-based payment or pay for performance.[1] The leadership skills needed here include decisiveness, an ability to get buy-in from stakeholders, adapt to a rapidly changing business landscape, and deliver results consistently.[2] As you can see all of these skills require considerable business acumen. When all is said and done, this is ALL human behavior. This is what you have been doing all of your professional career only now you are doing this on a larger scale where the rewards are greater, and the stakes are higher.

SUMMARY

This chapter offers a behavioral analysis of leadership and describes many of the activities required of leaders at each stage of their career. Leadership in its simplest form involves one person working with other people that have been trained, directed, and *motivated* to engage in tasks they otherwise do not prefer. This is a simple, stripped-down definition but serves the purpose of allowing an analysis of what is often overblown in our culture. To get started as a leader, we advise observing successful leaders to see how they manage their employees. As you observe, analyze the effectiveness of what they do. One of the first types of leadership you will engage in on your first job is the supervision of RBTs and trainees. As a young professional, you can volunteer to carry out smaller company projects with a few employees to get your footing. Then try your hand at conducting a meeting with a few people, and eventually lead a larger group.

NOTES

1 www.aafp.org/about/policies/all/value-based-payment.html
2 https://hbr.org/2017/05/what-sets-successful-ceos-apart

FOR FURTHER READING

de Bono, E. (2008). *Creativity workout: 62 exercises to unlock your most creative ideas*. Berkeley, CA: Ulysses Press.

Gottfredson, M., & Schaubert, S. (2008). *The breakthrough imperative: How the best managers get outstanding results*. New York: HarperCollins.

Rodel, J. (2021). *She thinks like a boss: Leadership. 9 essential skills for new female leaders in business & the workplace*. SC: Amazon Publications.

Wisdom, J. P. (2020). *Millennials' guide to management & leadership*. Winding Pathways Books.

REFERENCES

Daniels, A., & Bailey, J. (2014). *Performance management: Changing behavior that drives organizational effectiveness* (5th ed.). Atlanta: Performance Management Publications.

Daniels, A. C., & Daniels, J. E. (2005). *Measure of a leader: An actionable formula for legendary leadership*. Atlanta, GA: Performance Management.

Jurgens, H., Cordova, K., & Cruz, Y. (2021). *The ABA supervision handbook: A guide to quality fieldwork experience*. Ormond Beach, FL: WND Press.

Wooden, J., & Jamison, S. (2005). *Wooden on leadership*. New York: McGraw-Hill.

8

Assertiveness

If you don't have a seat at the table, you're probably on the menu.

—Elizabeth Warren

I was called into the clinical director's office as soon as I arrived at work. "I have two new cases for you, Angela," she said in an exasperated tone. "I know you are the one to step up here and help out . . ." The director's phone rang at that moment, and she waved me out of the room. This meant that I now had 17 cases to manage along with two BCaBAs and eight RBTs. I was beginning to collapse under the workload but didn't know how to tell her "No." I quietly crept out of the office and back to my cubicle.

Unfortunately, this is an all-too-common scenario in our field—too much work and too few people to pick up the load. The *cause* is largely a systems problem (to be discussed in more detail in Chapter 24) but the impact on caring, hardworking behavior analysts can be reduced by understanding the role of assertiveness in their day-to-day interactions with supervisors.

FRESH OUT OF GRAD SCHOOL, FIRST JOB

Most graduate programs in ABA do not teach assertiveness or even talk about it. We surmise that it is not in the faculty's best interest since they want students to accept their assigned homework,

DOI: 10.4324/9781003265573-10

papers, and presentations as valid learning experiences and complete them without asking questions. The power dynamic between students and faculty crushes any tendency to resist the academic and practicum work assigned. The net result is that when they take off their caps and gowns and take that first career step, new graduates are often woefully unprepared to engage in the necessary assertiveness to be successful in their first jobs.

There are basically three ways to react when your rights are infringed upon or you are treated with disrespect: you can be **passive, aggressive, or assertive** (Verderber, Macgeorge, Verderber, & Pruim, 2016, p. 297). People who avoid conflict, don't want to offend the other person, or are afraid of the outcome if they do, will naturally take the passive route as the easy way out (Smith, 2018, p. 4) as Angela did in our scenario above. While this may reduce any immediate negative reaction, the long-term effects will clearly be harmful and likely to lead to ***passive-aggressive behavior***, insomnia, substance abuse, high blood pressure as well as fatigue, and eventually resignation, a.k.a. burnout syndrome (Mayo Clinic, 2021).

Alternatively, some people naturally engage in ***aggressive responses*** when they are snubbed, opposed, or disputed. This reaction may be intermittently reinforced but the long-term effect in almost any work setting will be a reputation as someone who is "difficult," problematic, or "not a team player" (Smith, 2018, pp. 5–6).

> Being assertive requires an in-depth knowledge of the people with whom you are dealing, and it is appropriate only under specific circumstances. Knowing how and when to be assertive is a critical skill for effective behavior analysts.

Assertiveness 101

Using an assertive approach is difficult for behavior analysts who don't have experience in playing what is commonly referred to in the corporate world as "hardball." Assertiveness can be risky. Being assertive requires an in-depth knowledge of the people with whom you are dealing, and it is appropriate only under specific circumstances. Knowing how and when to be assertive is a critical skill for effective behavior analysts. Assertive communications should be direct and respectful, descriptive, involve appropriate body language, and preserve the relationship (Verderber et al., 2016, p. 300).

Interviewing For Your First Job

The first opportunity for you to apply your assertiveness skills will likely be when you are interviewing for your first full-time behavior analysis position. After narrowing down your options (Bailey & Burch, 2022. See Chapter 14: *Finding an Ethical Place to Work*), you will probably meet with a recruiter. If that goes well, you may have another meeting with a member of the administration of the company, and then finally with a behavior analyst who is possibly the clinical director (this sequence will vary with the size of the company). Assuming you are still interested, you will want to convey this with your questions and your body language, turn toward your interviewer, make good eye contact, be alert, listen closely and "keep a warm facial expression" (Smith, 2018, pp. 51–52). In terms of questions, the primary issues you should be concerned about are your working conditions (caseload, supervisees, required billable hours per week, who you will report to, their stand on the BACB ethics code, and their position on client rights and welfare, and any extra duties expected of BCBAs). You may want to avoid being a 1099 consultant because you will not be an employee and will not be entitled to any benefits such as the health insurance that is offered by the company. You will have to calculate and make your own tax payments quarterly and you will have to pay a self-employment tax.

The First 90 Days

The initial 90 days on a new job most often come with an unwritten grace period where you can ask questions that will later appear to be in the category of "stupid questions," but in the beginning are considered appropriate for a newbie. So, your first act of assertiveness at your new job will be to ask a lot of questions about how the organization works and exactly what is expected of you. If someone asks you to do something that you are not sure of, begin by being assertive. Say, "I don't understand," and then rephrase what has been asked of you to see if this results in a better description. When you are asking questions about a request that has been made of you, you'll want to have a very steady tone to your voice. Don't sound whiny or like you are trying to get out of something—you just want a clear understanding of what is expected. This is a time when you can ask about the table of the organization so you can understand what the power structure is within the organization.

Your first act of assertiveness at your new job will be to ask a lot of questions about how the organization works and exactly what is expected of you.

Learning to say "no" is a critical part of assertiveness for any behavior analyst.

Just Say "No"

Learning to say "no" is a critical part of assertiveness for any behavior analyst. Our interviews with behavior analysts from around the country indicate that saying "no" is one of the most difficult skills to develop, especially for new, young behavior analysts who are understandably eager to please their new employers.

One new behavior analyst we talked with described his frustration at a treatment program for clients with head injuries. It seems that he was led to believe that the orientation of the program was thoroughly behavioral. It soon became clear, however, that the staff wanted him to sign off on "canned" programs that came from a database of programs for previous clients. The behavior analyst wanted to do individualized functional assessments but was told, "We already know the cause of the behavior. Just plug in his name, and sign at the bottom." When he used his assertiveness skills and said "no," the administration fired him during his probation period without cause. About six months later, the facility closed after an investigation pertaining to its billing practices and data falsification.

Please Explain Yourself

Sometimes to say "no" you'll want to *include an explanation.* For example, when someone invites you to a work-related social event, you can decline the invitation politely. This "no" includes an explanation such as, "Thank you so much for inviting me, but I will be out of town that weekend," or "Thank you so much for inviting me, but I have young children, and I really like to stay home on the weekends."

If you are asked by someone to do something you simply don't have time to do, it is perfectly acceptable to let the person know you are busy: "I'd love to do training for your staff, but I am fully committed to doing three major projects for the next several months."

If you are good at what you do, people will begin to count on you as someone who can get the job done. Then you may find yourself getting requests to work on projects that are not within your skill set. One way to turn down a request for services you are not trained to provide is to say, "Thanks, John, I really appreciate your support, but I don't think I am the best person to lead this particular project. I really don't have any experience working with adult offenders."

As a treatment team member, you will find many times when you have to say "no" to a roomful of professionals: "With all due respect to Janice, I believe her suggestion that sensory stimulation should be the major focus of treatment is not the way we want to go. There is no data to support this approach as a means of reducing maladaptive behaviors. The first logical step here is to conduct a functional analysis." This is the "no" you will use to *advocate the use of sound behavioral procedures* that are based on science.

Ask for What You Want

Another major aspect of assertiveness is *asking for what you want.* If you don't ask, you probably won't get what you need or want, because whoever is making the decisions can't read your mind and doesn't know what is important to you. Requests such as asking for an occasional day off or a chance to go to an annual state or national behavioral conference might be granted, especially if you are highly valued for your creative ideas and you make your requests well in advance.

How am I Doing?

Another form of assertiveness is asking for frequent feedback on how you are doing. Although this might seem like fishing for reinforcers or asking for trouble, regular feedback can help you improve your own performance. Far too often, it is company policy that you will receive an annual performance review. As behaviorists, we know that receiving feedback at the end of a year for something you did 11 months ago is much too delayed to have any effect. Don't be a pest but asking for feedback at least quarterly is a form of assertiveness that will pay off in the long run. If your supervisor does not want to take the time to put the feedback in writing, you can summarize your meeting and send the notes in an email to your supervisor so there will be a paper trail. By requesting frequent feedback, you can show your supervisors that you have a strong desire to be an excellent employee. This will put you in good stead when you must occasionally say "no" to a request.

Assertiveness On Behalf Your Client

One of the most frequent occasions for you to be assertive is when a group decision is to be made and you have input as the behavior analyst. In team meetings, there will be many times when someone in the group will be pushing for action that in your opinion is not warranted. As you listen closely, you might determine that because this person has taken a very strong position and has presented it in an adamant, emotional manner, everyone is inclined to just go along. People often go along with a bad plan simply because it is the easiest thing to do. Furthermore, there will be some people at the table who are motivated by thoughts such as, "Why rock the boat and slow everything down?" "If we hurry, we can go to lunch sooner," or "I don't want to make this woman mad; I have to work with her at several schools." As an ethical behavior analyst, before you decide it is time to be assertive on an issue, *make sure that you are right* and that your proposal to the group will improve the client's well-being. Remember, to be effective you can't be assertive on *every* single issue, only on a few. Make sure this is *the issue* you are willing to push.

YOUNG PROFESSIONAL (3–5 YEARS)

Training Supervisees

Once you have settled into your first job and are known around the company as a team player and a client advocate, you can turn your assertiveness skills to larger issues. This might include working with your supervisees to help them become more assertive regarding the handling of clients who are either trying to become too friendly or those who are at the opposite end of the continuum. For the former, you will need to model for the supervisee how to say "No, I'm sorry. I'm not allowed to babysit for you on the weekends," or, "I really appreciate the offer, but no I can't go with you to Walt Disney World®. I will help you prepare for this big event though, let me talk with my supervisor about how to do that . . ."

> **It is not well known, but many behavior techs and RBTs often suffer insults, threats, and abuse at the hands of family members.**

It is not well known but many behavior techs and RBTs often suffer insults, threats, and abuse at the hands of family members. These junior but very significant members of our profession simply do not deserve to be treated this way, and their first line of defense should be to assert themselves and then immediately report the encounter to you, their supervisor. Modeling for them an appropriate way to respond at the first instance there is a problem gives supervisees dignity and lets them know that they are valued.

Assertiveness in Meetings

When you are ready to assert yourself in a meeting, you'll have to do several things simultaneously. First, sit up straight, put your hands in front of you on the table, and calmly fold them. When it is your turn, present your information in a logical, organized, and concise fashion. When you do this, people are likely to agree with you. But sometimes there will be another professional who does not agree and, furthermore, who thinks their approach is the only one to consider. This is when you will need to use your very best assertiveness skills. Make good, strong eye contact with the person who is bullying the group into their way of thinking. In your own words, say something that basically conveys the following message: "With all due respect to Tan, I have to say I disagree with what is being proposed here. I'm concerned that (client name) is not being well served by what we are about to do. Here are some problems with this approach . . ."

If you aren't successful after explaining why you think the recommended approach presents problems, you may have to be a little more assertive: "I can't agree with our moving forward with this. It appears to me that what you are about to decide is to use the solution requiring the least effort. The easy way is not the right way in this case. Let's slow this process down and reconsider our options."

As you speak, move your gaze from one person to the next at the table. Do not raise your voice, do not go shrill, and don't squint, roll your eyes, emit loud groans of exasperation, or make faces. By all means, do *not* apologize for what you are saying. Then re-present your strategy for the solution, the right solution, to the group. Start by using your DRO (differential reinforcement of other behaviors) skills to identify those parts of the decision with which you do agree. Emphasize how your plan benefits your client. Stay with this message, and do not go off course and talk about other benefits.

MID-CAREER (6–10 YEARS)

Now that you are well established in the company, are well known as a smart, successful person who means to protect client rights, can solve problems, and on occasion can be assertive when you are passionate about something, you will be looking to make a difference on a different level. At this stage of your career, you may see an opportunity to take the company in a new direction by offering behavioral services to a new client population or perhaps open a new clinic in a rapidly expanding part of the state. Your senior decision-makers on the board of directors may be more conservative on such matters, and you will now have to dust off your assertiveness skills once again. The skills themselves are not new. They are just applied on a larger scale. For example, you may have to assert yourself with the city planning commission, an architect, or a commercial builder. By now you should have some years behind you of successful "Wins" by being assertive so you will be operating from a strong position with a good history of reinforcement. A lot is at stake in promoting initiatives like this so make sure that you have done your research and your due diligence.

> As a senior, respected member of the company, you will no doubt spend most of your time in meetings where your assertiveness will be essential to the success of your company as you try and guide it toward a bright future.

SENIOR BEHAVIOR ANALYST

With a decade or more of experience, it is highly likely that you will have been promoted to senior vice president, CEO, or president of the company where you started your career. At this level, your direct work with clients is behind you and there is an expectation that you will be applying your behavior analysis skills, including assertiveness, to manage the company, delegate routine assignments to junior associates, advance the corporate agenda, and influence members of the board in setting policy. You will be handling funding and trying to predict the future of our behavior analysis "industry." As a senior, respected member of the company, you will no doubt spend most of your time in meetings where your assertiveness will be essential to the success of your company as you try and guide it toward a bright future.

SUMMARY

This chapter describes how the essential skill of being assertive is applied through the four stages of one's career. Fresh out of graduate school and on their first jobs, behavior analysts must learn to avoid a passive or aggressive stance when dealing with people. The most successful posture is one of assertiveness. This involves a steady tone of voice and corresponding appropriate body language that exudes confidence and captures the attention of the audience. Using assertiveness to protect clients' rights, advance a worthy position, or promote an agenda engenders trust and produces consensus which allows for smoother decision-making. As a new BCBA, you will no doubt have many requests and opportunities thrust at you, and learning to say, "No" to some of these will be essential to the development of a manageable workload. Being assertive on behalf of your clients and your supervisees will be essential to their well-being and their progress.

FOR FURTHER READING

Detz, J. (2000). *It's not what you say, it's how you say it.* New York: St. Martin's Griffin.

McQuain, J. (1996). *Power language: Getting the most out of your words.* New York: Houghton Mifflin.

Pachter, B., & Magee, S. (2000). *The power of positive confrontation.* New York: Marlowe.

Skinner, B. F. (1957). *Verbal behavior.* Englewood, NJ: Prentice-Hall.

REFERENCES

Bailey, J. S., & Burch, M. R. (2022). *Ethics for behavior analysts* (4th ed.). New York: Routledge, Inc.

Mayo Clinic. (2021). *Job burnout: How to spot it and take action*. Retrieved from www.mayoclinic.org/healthy-lifestyle/adult-health/in-depth/burnout/art-20046642

Smith, S. R. (2018). *5 Steps to assertiveness*. Berkley, CA: Althea Press.

Verderber, K. S., Macgeorge, E. L., Verderber, R. F., & Pruim, D. E. (2016). *Interact: Interpersonal communication concepts, skills and contexts* (14th ed.). New York: Oxford University Press.

9

Cultural Responsiveness

Every person needs a place that is furnished with hope.

—Maya Angelou

FRESH OUT OF GRAD SCHOOL, FIRST JOB

This new chapter in the *25 Skills* text was prompted by the 2020 BACB Ethics Code for Behavior Analysts which requires that behavior analysts, "acquire knowledge and skills related to cultural responsiveness and diversity."[1] This information along with an additional requirement for BCBAs to "evaluate their own biases" and demonstrate their ability to meet the needs of their clients who may have varied backgrounds makes it clear that this is an indispensable part of the successful behavior analyst's repertoire. Depending on where you went to school and where you received your supervision, you may have had a rich and challenging experience where you came away with new insights into your own biases. You might have also developed a strong skill set for active engagement with clients from other cultures or with very different backgrounds than yours. However, this may not have been your experience. If you have limited experience with the cultures and backgrounds of others, on your first job you have some serious catching up to do. All behavior analysts should get to know,

DOI: 10.4324/9781003265573-11

appreciate, and truly value people from a different status in terms of their "age, disability, ethnicity, gender expression/identity, immigration status, marital/relationship status, national origin, race, religion, sexual orientation, or socioeconomic status."[2]

What *is* important is that you know how the family in front of you operates and what is important to *them*.

Learning About the Client

Learning how to interact with individuals from all these categories could be an overwhelming task, however, from a practical point of view the actual requirement is that you meet the needs of the clients assigned to you. This will be a subset of the above, so the initial task related to your job comes down to getting to know three or four families, and professionals with whom you work that have backgrounds or cultures different than yours. However, we talk often about aggressive curiosity (Chapter 25 of this book), and we believe that truly getting to know where a person is coming from can make you a better person. Read about different cultures, talk to people who aren't clients, and have them educate you and help you gain a deeper understanding of people and cultures different than you. You will be better off for it and your life will be so much richer.

As mentioned previously, it is not a requirement that to meet a client's needs you must know the *complete* history of their culture (e.g., when their religion began), understand the origins and significance of each tradition, and be fluent in the traditional family hierarchy, food preferences, taboos, and religious practices. What *is* important is that you know how the client or family in front of you operates and what is important to *them*. This makes the task more doable but does require additional competencies which we covered previously in Chapter 2: *Interpersonal communications*.

Primary among these are effective, active listening skills, a desire to learn everything you can about this person or family, and an ability to accommodate their preferences (See also Chapter 2 of this book). This may require some give and take by both parties since the individual or families will at the same time be learning about behavior analysis—minus the jargon—and they should want to put *their* best foot forward to receive optimal service from their behavior analysis team.

Your safest bet is to double or triple the time you would normally spend getting to know about a family's habits, hobbies, food, fun preferences, where they work, what they do, and what their expectations are for behavioral services.

Even if you have extensively studied the culture of your clients or read case studies about individuals from some of these diverse backgrounds, you should not assume you can generalize any of this to the client that is sitting across from you. Your safest bet is to double or triple the time you would normally spend getting to know about a family's habits, hobbies, food, fun preferences, where they work, what they do, and what their expectations are for behavioral services.

Dr. Noor Syed and her students (Syed et al., 2020) have suggested a few topics to discuss and questions you may want to ask to get acquainted with your new client so you can develop a behavior plan that meets their needs and that they will support. This list is adapted from their recommendations.

- FAMILY INFORMATION/PREFERENCES
  - Please tell me about your family.
  - What are some common family activities?
  - What are your daily and weekly routines?
  - How would you like me to communicate with you (in person, phone call, text)?
  - Which language is predominantly used at home?
  - In which language would you like me to teach your child?

    - How would you like to be addressed?
    - Is there anything else you'd like me to know about your family?
- SERVICES, IN-HOME
    - What are your expectations for services?
    - Specific times of day therapy cannot be given.
    - How would you describe your ideal therapist?
    - Specific times of day therapy cannot be given.
    - Gender preference for therapists?
    - What is your preferred gender pronoun?
- SERVICES, IN-CLINIC
    - Are there materials and activities to avoid?
    - What are times you can work and not work?
    - How will you get to and from work?
    - Have you made arrangements to come to our clinic?
    - Do you need flexible scheduling time?
    - Are there specific accommodations you would prefer (i.e., gender neutral bathroom, nursing room)?

As you go through these items, you will be taking notes and asking follow-up questions to make sure you understand their responses and the implications for your treatment plan and your behavioral team.

Following this gathering of information, you will want to go over the Declaration of *Professional Practices and Procedures* for Behavior Analysts (see Chapter 13 in Bailey & Burch, 2022) for details. The BACB now refers to a document such as this as the Service Agreement (Code 3.04) to make sure the parents/caregivers/stakeholders have a good understanding of how behavior analysis works, what the limitations are, and their requirements for cooperation and implementation (i.e., parent/caregiver training). What you expect from them should be very clear in the beginning so that there are no misunderstandings later about their commitment to the forthcoming behavior change plan.

Applying What You've Learned

With all the information you have accumulated, the next step is to put together a behavior plan unique to this client or family. The plan should delineate any limitations and preferences. It should also consider their expectations for behavioral outcomes as well as their involvement in the process that is about to commence. This is not an easy task; it requires sensitivity to client needs as well as a thorough understanding of behavioral principles and procedures. Expect mid-course corrections based on the incoming data and regular feedback you will be receiving.

On your first job, you may be expected to not only conduct these interviews and develop these client-centric plans but train others to do so as well. If your agency has not already done this, you may want to see if you can arrange monthly meetings of staff and administrators on the topic of cultural responsiveness where everyone may share experiences with various populations. You can bring in invited speakers to address certain populations or issues of concern.

YOUNG PROFESSIONAL (3–5 YEARS)

At this point, you are an experienced professional. Interacting with and providing services to a variety of individuals from different cultures and backgrounds should be second nature. Cultural responsiveness should be well ingrained into your repertoire, and you should be prepared to acquire even more knowledge about the cultures of your clients. This is known as cultural humility (Hook, Davis, Owen, Worthington, & Utsey, 2013) and it will make you even more effective. Periodically check in with your clients to make sure they are satisfied with the cultural responsiveness of the RBTs and other members of the behavior analysis team. Consider exploring and interacting with

> **Being in a leadership position means that you can move your company policies in ways not possible earlier in your career.**

people of other cultures in your community to increase your understanding of the diverse backgrounds that exist there.

MID-CAREER (6–10 YEARS)

Given the many people from different backgrounds that they have worked with, the mid-career behavior analyst should have a strong sense of cultural responsiveness. With six to ten years of experience, you are in the position to have a greater impact on the services being delivered by your agency. Being in a leadership position means that you can move your company policies in ways not possible earlier in your career. You can include requirements for specific training in cultural responsiveness (including Diversity, Equity, and Inclusion training, Chapter 13) by all your behavioral staff. The occasional guest speaker can be upgraded as a more permanent part of the in-service program as you push for more diversity in your organization. The latter may involve recruiting young people to become RBTs and launching a broader search for BCBAs of diverse backgrounds. Whereas once you had to hire translators to work with your BCBAs, this now may be less necessary if you have behavior analysts who are linguistically diverse on your staff.

SENIOR BEHAVIOR ANALYST

Many disadvantaged populations suffer from not only poverty and illiteracy but also chronic illness. Some of your clients may be in this situation. As the owner, clinical director, or chair of the board of directors, you could lead an initiative to have your company more involved in community efforts to ameliorate these conditions in your community (Levy & Sidel, 2006). As a leader in your organization, you may be able to advance cultural responsiveness in broader ways in your community. One way would be to include "resilience" in behavior programming. As described by Miller, Cruz, and Shahla (2019) this refers to "behaviors that enable families to cope more effectively and emerge hardier from crises or persistent stresses." See also Hawley and DeHaan (1996) for descriptions of behaviors that families could acquire to help them cope including dealing with and surviving stressful situations, and adapting behavioral responses to changing economic and environmental conditions.

SUMMARY

This chapter describes the vital role that cultural responsiveness plays in the design and delivery of behavioral services to clients who may be of a different cultural background or status than the behavior analyst. It is important to learn as much about your client as you can on the front end of services and to have the client participate in the design of your proposed behavior plan before it is implemented. This can be accomplished by engaging all your interpersonal communications skills and asking probing questions of the client or family as to their preferences, expectations for services, and any limitations that might need to be accommodated. It is important that you make any changes that need to be made, and that you keep in close touch with the client/family throughout the treatment process to make sure that they continue to be satisfied with their services.

NOTES

1 BACB Ethics Code for Behavior Analysts 2022, Code 1.07.
2 BACB Ethics Code for Behavior Analysts 2022, Code 1.07.

FOR FURTHER READING

Conners, B. M., & Capell, S. T. (Eds.). (2021) *Multiculturalism and diversity in applied behavior analysis: Bridging theory and application.* New York: Routledge, Inc.

REFERENCES

Bailey, J. S., & Burch, M. R. (2022). *Ethics for behavior analysts* (4th ed.). New York: Routledge, Inc.

Hawley, D. R., & DeHaan, L. (1996). Toward a definition of family resilience: Integrating lifespan and family perspectives. *Family Process*, *35*(3), 283–298. https://doi.org/10.1111/j.1545-5300.1996.00283.x

Hook, J. N., Davis, D. E., Owen, J., Worthington, E. L., & Utsey, S. O. (2013). Cultural humility: Measuring openness to culturally diverse clients. *Journal of Counseling Psychology*, *60*(3), 353–366. https://doi. org/10.1037/a0032595

Levy, B. S., & Sidel, V. W. (2006). *The nature of social injustice and its impact on public health*. Oxford: Oxford University Press.

Miller, K. L., Cruz, R. A., & Shahla, A. R. (2019). Inherent tensions and possibilities: Behavior analysis and cultural responsiveness. *Behavior and Social Issues*. Association for Behavior Analysis International, *28*, 203. https://doi.org/10.1007/s42822-019-00013-y

Syed, N., Allgood, A., Gayle, R., Piazza, J., Orland, N., Rohrer, J., & Suzio, C. (2020). *Lecture 2: Culture, cultural humility, and cultural competence (PowerPoint slides)*. Beverly, MA: Van Loan School at Endicott College.

10

Client Advocate

The best way to find yourself is to lose yourself in the service of others.

—Mahatma Gandhi

The traditional role of the BCBA is that of a technician who is an expert in the technology of behavior change (Miltenberger, 2016), with a strong background in the science of behavior (Skinner, 1953). Technicians apply what they know about behavior analysis to problems that are referred to them by a client directly or by the company for which they work. However, with the advent of the Behavior Analyst Certification Board in 1999, the role evolved and expanded from technician to professional. This is someone who knows how to change behavior and who is also required to follow a strict code of ethics that includes responsibility for the welfare of their client (Bailey & Burch, 2021). Thus, this adds the additional role of *Advocate.* Advocates act in favor of others. In behavioral settings, advocacy means making recommendations for treatments and supporting the rights of clients.

FRESH OUT OF GRAD SCHOOL, FIRST JOB

As a brand new BCBA, you will have a chance to train your team of behavior analysts to not only be good behavior techs but also

DOI: 10.4324/9781003265573-12

advocates for the clients that you serve. You will be positioned to discuss clients' rights with them on a regular basis in your group meetings and to review them regularly on an individual basis during regular supervision sessions. Here is another example from a question that came into the ABA Ethics Hotline:

> I currently provide services to a client in a group home setting. The client usually asks for a glass of water once every couple of hours. She typically drinks the entire glass in one sitting, rather than taking sips. Over the last couple of weeks, I have observed group home staff deny the client water, with the reasoning being that she had "already had water this afternoon" and that she had to wait until the next mealtime.

The BCBA's overall goal is to make a socially significant improvement in the life of the client.

This BCBA was working on other goals and just happened to make this observation during a supervision session. It is unquestionable that clients have a right to water (physicians recommend six glasses per day) and denying this basic right could not only be detrimental to their health but it may instigate other behavior problems as well. As an advocate, your role is to watch for such incidents and to take appropriate action. When contacted by the behavior analyst, the Hotline ethicist advised to start by meeting with the group home operator to see what could be done to correct this unfortunate situation. The phrase "maximize benefits" in Code 3.01 spells out an additional, subtle, requirement that this behavior analyst met while she was working on other goals requested by the family and the group-home stakeholder. Her observation will no doubt contribute to the welfare of her client above and beyond any success she has with behavioral goals and objectives. The BCBA's overall goal is to make a socially significant improvement in the life of the client. Here is one more example:

> My company, to increase billable hours, is mandating that all clients have a minimum of 20 hours per week of behavioral services and

> have specified that if they do not, services will be discontinued. Some of my clients, in my professional opinion, require only 10 hours and some require 15 hours per week. It seems unethical to meet this random number of hours just to increase the bottom line for investors.

In this case, the BCBA is *advocating* for the "appropriate amount and level of behavioral service provision and oversight required to meet defined client goals" as specified in Code 3.12, although the company has a different objective. A somewhat different challenge is represented by this question that came from a student in the first-author's ethics class:

> I was assigned to work as an RBT with a 5-year-old in the home. When I arrived, I was struck by the lack of cleanliness and an odor that smelled like cat urine. The only place I could work with the client was on the living room couch (after removing pizza boxes, plastic soda cups and cigarette butts). I had been given a behavior plan for manding with the child but was immediately distracted by his scratching and itching and then found myself doing the same. I cut the session short. When I got to my car, I found that I had flea bites around my legs and ankles. I called my supervisor and told her that I'm not going back until the home is cleaned up and suitable for therapy.

In this case, the BCBA needed to advocate for better living conditions for this child and may end up operating as a mandated reporter in a call to the health department if the parents cannot make the necessary improvements to the living conditions for this child. Here is an equally difficult recent situation.

> I just found out that one of our very difficult in-home clients is locked in her bare bedroom at night. She sleeps on a mattress on the floor. There is nothing for her to play with except for two plush animals with the stuffing missing.

In this case, if the behavior analyst is not successful in getting the parents to consider a safer and more humane arrangement for their child at night, it may be time to take their advocacy to a higher level, i.e., the mandated reporter requirements also mentioned in and contact CPS (child protective services).

YOUNG PROFESSIONAL (3–5 YEARS)

Once you complete your first few years as a behavior analyst, you will be able to establish yourself as a role model for advocacy for clients. You will oversee your treatment teams and have a routine worked out for training all your RBTs, trainees, and BCaBAs on what to watch for as they conduct their therapy sessions. As a more seasoned BCBA, you may have difficult cases transferred to you from other behavior analysts and this will give you an opportunity to do a top-down review of the cases. This is the time to closely examine not only the appropriateness and effectiveness of the behavior plan but also clients' rights issues. Are the clients assigned the appropriate "amount and level" of behavioral services? Are there any mitigating circumstances such as environmental or medical conditions that are affecting the client's ability to benefit from the treatment? Does the plan meet current requirements for best practice? Does there need to be a placement review? If the client is showing success, is there a program fading and seamless discharge plan in place? Here is an example of a medical condition that would benefit from advocacy and strong support from the behavior analyst.

> I am a BCBA in a school district. We have a student who had a brain tumor removed a few years ago and was diagnosed with TBI following that surgery. He has a shunt, some vision loss, and loss of mobility. A recent evaluation conducted by the school district shows regression across all areas—cognitive, behavior, etc. Since returning from his most recent surgery, the aggression has escalated in both frequency and intensity. The student is now in a self-contained high school classroom. The situation is getting extremely dangerous as he has hurt multiple staff and students. Adults and peers are very afraid of him. I have advocated for the student's placement to be changed to a special alternate setting that could handle his aggression AND his medical needs, but

have been met with resistance by the administration. At this point, I am quite concerned that someone is going to be seriously harmed, especially if he remains in the current setting. Due to his medical condition, increased aggression, and cognitive regression, I am questioning if ABA will be effective in reducing his aggression even under optimal environmental conditions. Is it possible ABA may not work for this student due to the behavior being a manifestation of a medical condition?

Using your experience as an advocate, you may be able to establish an *advocacy committee* at your school that reviews difficult cases and makes recommendations for the action to be taken.

MID-CAREER (6–10 YEARS)

At this stage in your career, you will be in a position to have some influence with client advocacy in your agency, company, or association. Using your experience as an advocate, you may be able to establish an *advocacy committee* at your school that reviews difficult cases and makes recommendations for the action to be taken. Conducting an internal review of all client cases to determine the most frequent client rights violations that are encountered would be a good first step. To emphasize the advocacy role that all staff should have, you may consider inviting someone from the Abuse Hotline to give a presentation on what constitutes client abuse and neglect and how to proceed if you find a client that meets these legal requirements.

SENIOR BEHAVIOR ANALYST

In your capacity as a senior member of your management team, you may have an opportunity to impact the company's policies regarding advocacy for clients of the agency. Some companies are designating a director-level staff as the client advocate or if they are large enough, they are hiring a person to work independently in that capacity full time. The goal is for one person to be the voice of the client if they feel the client has been slighted in their treatment or an inappropriate number of hours is assigned. This was demonstrated in the case earlier where services would be discontinued if the therapists did not increase their hours to a minimum of 20 hours per week. Here is another example where a client advocate would clearly be needed.

> My two sons were receiving ABA services from your company. Services started six months ago, and I am not happy about recent events. The therapist was very unprofessional initially. She did not show up on time or give my children the full hours they were scheduled for. Some weeks she came just two out of five days—then she stopped coming altogether. After that, I contacted her supervisor who said she would meet with me to discuss the matter. Three days later she showed up and said that the therapist just quit, and she did not have a replacement. My children have now been without services for going on two months. Do I need to take legal action on this matter?

This case demonstrates the need for a senior-level member of the firm to act as a client advocate who can step in, take charge, and solve problems. An investigation obviously is in order, some personnel changes may be necessary, consumer-service training must be instituted, and new policies established to avoid this charade from happening in the future.

SUMMARY

This chapter presented the case for behavior analysts acting as advocates for their clients. This role, along with being mandated reporters, is mentioned in the BACB Ethics Code. While they are primarily involved with developing behavior-change programs, behavior analysts must be prepared to look for other variables that may be operating such as the physical or medical condition of the client or causal factors in the environment. Supporting clients' rights is a big part of being an advocate. Behavior analysts should be constantly on guard for violations of those rights. This includes ensuring that clients receive the correct amount and type of service. It also ensures the proper implementation of the plan as written and the introduction of goals that will improve the client's quality of life and maximize their potential. BCBAs need to be knowledgeable of and aware of medical issues and be prepared to recommend a medical consultation if there is any hint of a biological cause of a behavior. As behavior analysts grow in experience, they may begin to expand the realm of advocacy services for their clients including becoming a dedicated, independent advocate who can take charge and solve service-delivery problems.

REFERENCES

Bailey, J. S., & Burch, M. R. (2021). *The RBT® ethics code: Mastering the BACB ethics code for registered behavior technicians.* New York: Routledge, Inc.

Miltenberger, R. G. (2016). *Behavior modification: Principles and procedures* (6th ed.). Boston: Cengage Learning.

Skinner, B. F. (1953). *Science and human behavior.* New York: MacMillan Company.

Unit Three

Applying Your Behavioral Knowledge

The owners of a multi-state ABA company were getting ready to evaluate staff and develop improvement plans. They discussed a BCBA who had been on the job for five years.

Owner 1 started by saying the BCBA had excellent clinical skills and was "so good" with clients.

Owner 2 replied, "I believe there are some serious problems here. At five years out, we expect to see BCBAs who can use behavioral procedures such as shaping and PM to get results in any setting from schools to the clinic, including all our sites.

DOI: 10.4324/9781003265573-13

By now, this BCBA should be a pro at handling difficult people, but she's not. I know there is a behavioral approach to this—why is she not using it?

And another thing, BCBAs are professionals, and they are required to adhere to their Code including following the principles of DEI in their daily work. She's not always doing this."

11

Managing Difficult People

What you allow is what will continue.

—Anonymous

Anyone who is employed long enough will encounter people who are difficult. "Difficult," of course, means different things to different people. Difficult people are trying, challenging, problematic, and can be tiring. They are hard to manage, and they make things hard for the people around them. In the case of the behavior analyst, a difficult person is someone who slows down or derails our attempt to effectively implement our behavior-change agenda which can range from an individual client's behavior program to the reimagination of a large corporation.

You'll notice in this chapter that we use commonly recognized labels such as *lazy*, *defiant*, or *self-centered*. We do this because these words can immediately conjure up a vivid image for the reader. In the work setting, however, as a behavior analyst, you'll have to quickly move beyond labels and any emotions you are feeling, put on your behavior analyst hat, and begin looking at *observable, measurable behaviors*, and their causes to manage a difficult person.

Difficult people have a wide variety of behaviors and responses that make them difficult. Opposing new ideas, resisting feedback, misrepresenting responsibility for a work product, being

DOI: 10.4324/9781003265573-14

manipulative, undermining and sabotaging others, bullying, lying, dramatizing every issue, complaining, not meeting deadlines, refusing to follow protocols, criticizing others and their work, arguing about everything, pointing out why any new suggestion will not work, actually causing problems so they can appear to be the hero who solves them, and refusing to help, as in "It's not my job," are just some of the characteristics that can be seen in difficult people. These are people who prevent a department from being calm, organized, reinforcing, and effective. They can push good workers over the edge and make them angry, frustrated, or depressed. They can derail projects and kill morale.

The nature of the working relationship you have with the difficult individual or where the person is on the organizational chart has a great deal to do with how you will approach this problem. If you are pitching an idea to the vice president of manufacturing for a new incentive system and you encounter resistance, this person might be difficult in a way that is totally different from the way a colleague criticizes your fashion choice or how you trim your beard. If you supervise a BCaBA who is a constant complainer, turns in sloppy work, or is always late in submitting their billable hours, this presents a different kind of difficulty.

Problematic and challenging people are found at all levels in your organization and the community as well; it is important for you to be able to deal with clients, stakeholders, co-workers, and administrators all the way up to the CEO.

FRESH OUT OF GRAD SCHOOL, FIRST JOB

"It's Almost All Verbal Behavior"

As soon as you begin your first job, it is important to set the stage for managing *difficult* people, i.e., those who make our lives difficult one way or another. Our analysis follows Skinner's lead (Skinner, 1957) in pointing out that these behaviors are more specifically *verbal* behaviors, which is to say that they are behaviors mediated by another person or several individuals. Categorizing them as verbal reminds us that since they are maintained by someone in the immediate environment, we can begin to look for *speaker-listener* relationships (Skinner, 1957, p. 11). Foremost among these is *stimulus control* (Skinner, 1957, p. 31) which establishes that certain people have become stimuli in the presence of which some challenging behavior is emitted, i.e., the person is an S^D. The next step in the sequence is to determine what reinforcer is maintaining the troublesome verbal behavior as shown in Figures 11.1, 11.2, and 11.3. We assume that the standard categories for functional analysis are operating here, i.e., attention from the listener or escape from some task presented by a speaker.

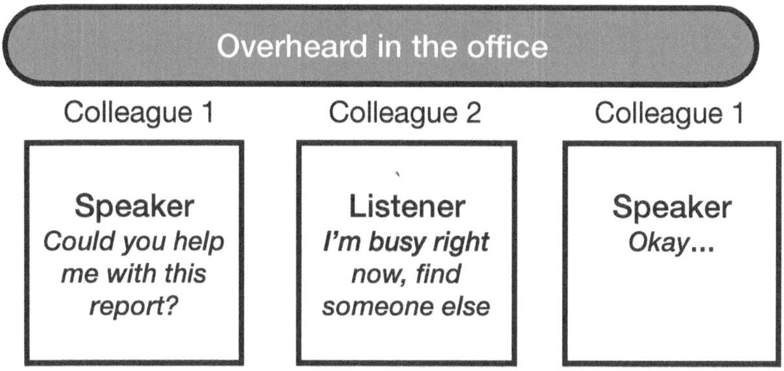

Figure 11.1 This figure shows how one colleague may reinforce a refusal to help another colleague.

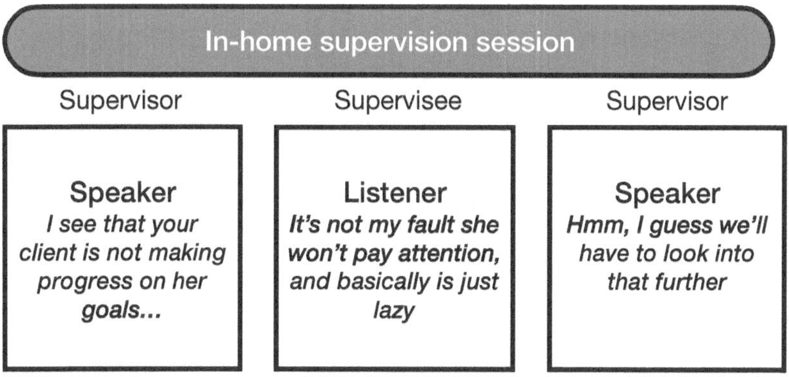

Figure 11.2 This figure shows how a supervisee may be accidentally reinforced by a supervisor for making excuses.

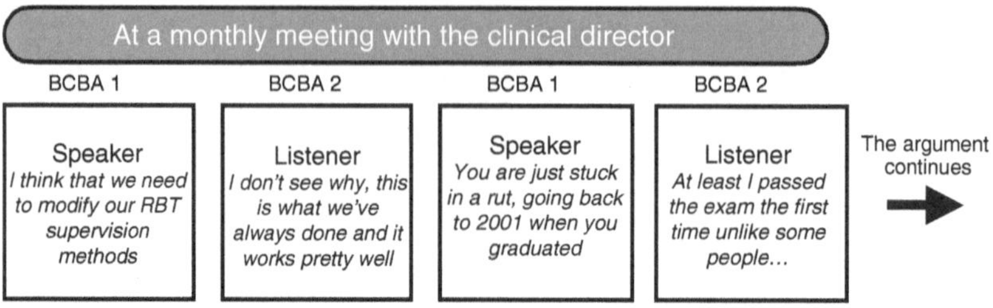

Figure 11.3 This figure shows how one BCBA may inadvertently reinforce another BCBA for getting off track and arguing.

Our Unique Position

As behavior analysts, we are in a unique position in any company or organization because we understand the concepts of reinforcement history, motivational operations, the "Circumstances View"[1] (Friman, 2021), as well as behavior-change methods such as behavior shaping, stimulus fading, behavioral momentum, and DRO (Michael, 2004), all of which are easily applied in any organization. Assuming you can apply the basic principles with your clients, it should not be too much of a stretch to use them with supervisees, colleagues, clients, and administrators. Beginning when you first get out of graduate school, you will need a willingness to test your skills with each of these groups.

Some Assumptions

As behavior analysts, we are prone to act when we see a behavior that needs to be modified. This could also apply when we encounter a consistently difficult person. If you have tried being reasonable, letting the person freely express themselves, and just plain avoiding them, you may decide to try your hand at nudging the difficult person toward more acceptable behavior. We assume that you *can* apply what you know about behavior change with clients to the adults in your environment and further that you are willing to do so. Some people can talk a good game but are not quite up to the task of applying contingencies with difficult grownups. One final requirement is that we strongly recommend reading, or re-reading Dale Carnegie's classic *How to Win Friends and Influence People* (Carnegie, 1981) Parts One to Three; his approach, written in layman's terms, fits well with our behavioral methodology and theory of behavior. A few of his key points include:

1. Smile
2. Don't criticize, condemn, or complain
3. Give honest and sincere appreciation
4. Become genuinely interested in other people
5. Encourage others to talk about themselves and be a good listener
6. Talk in terms of the other person's interests
7. Make the other person feel important—and do it sincerely

Controlling Variables

Before you start thinking about your behavior plan, you must try and determine what the controlling variables are. While at this level of your career, you cannot do a functional analysis, but you can approximate that by exercising your imagination and blending it with your personal experience to arrive at some good guesses. As described earlier, some of the variables involve social reinforcement, others are environmental, and still others involve contingencies of reinforcement. Here are some examples to think about.

Some Difficult *Behaviors*	***Maintained by . . .***
• Saying "Yes" but meaning "No"	• If they say "No" they will be punished.
• Arguing over trivial matters	• Arguing buys some time.
• Throwing up roadblocks	• Roadblocks cause distractions.
• Not following instructions	• Don't understand instructions, if they do they don't make sense, i.e., no rationale for them.
• Distracting you with crazy theories	• Clients/stakeholders are not science trained.
• Misrepresenting their actions	• Covering their tracks avoids punishment.

(Continued)

Some Difficult *Behaviors*	*Maintained by . . .*
• Disingenuous verbal behavior (lying)	• Lying has been reinforced since 1st grade (escape contingency).
• Putting convenience over ethics and profit over client treatment	• The company is owned by private equity and must show month-over-month profits.

Dealing With Clients & Stakeholders

Lack of Cooperation, Failure to Follow Through

One frequent complaint about dealing with families and stakeholders is that they do not follow through with behavior plans, are inconsistent in their applications, or in some cases, someone actually sabotages the behavior plan to ensure that it does not work. In order to negotiate these difficult behaviors, it is necessary to ask yourself some key questions about your relationship with the family.

Ask Yourself . . .	*What to Do*
• What is their history with the client?	• Conduct an informal FBA.
• Are your expectations appropriate?	• Adjust expectations based on MOs.
• Were they involved in choosing the goals?	• Set short term, measurable goals.
• Competing behaviors & obligations?	• Negotiate on these goals.
• What did your training of them look like?	• Invest in BST as your training model.
• Do you have a good working relationship with the family & stakeholders?	• Frequent meetings where you "take their temperature" to determine where you stand with them on trust, compassion, and competence.

Dealing With Supervisees

Poor Work Ethic, Making Excuses, Faking Data or Time Log

Many things can go wrong when you are working with new supervisees, trainees, or RBTs. This may be their first professional job and they may have problems with consistency, they may not understand the importance of taking data accurately or having quality interactions with clients or stakeholders. This is where you must understand the effects of the environment, pay scale, training, and many other variables which can produce unacceptable behavior of a supervisee.

> *A supervisor who is not there when needed can cause real anguish and make you wonder if you are appreciated and supported.*

Ask Yourself . . .	***What to Do***
• What is their work history? Previous supervision?	• Conduct an informal FBA on the problem behaviors.
• *Are your* expectations appropriate?	• Review your goals for each therapist and make sure they are appropriate
• Are they working with the type of client they are interested in?	• Can you assign them to different clients?
• Are the working conditions optimal for their participation? Hours? Pay? Time off?	• Review their assigned hours and pay scale to make sure it is competitive with other companies in the area.
• What did your training of them look like?	• Invest in BST as your training model for all trainees.
• Is your supervision consistent, oriented toward their professional improvement, client-oriented?	• Review your supervision methods to make sure they meet BACB Guidelines for amount of time, quality of training and feedback.

Dealing With Your Supervisor

Who Doesn't Respond to Your Email or Return Phone Calls

A supervisor who is not there when needed can cause real anguish and make you wonder if you are appreciated and supported. However, before you rush to judgment consider a few variables that might be controlling your supervisor's behavior.

Ask Yourself . . .	***What to Do***
• Are your expectations for your supervisor appropriate? • Are you too needy?	• Spend more 1:1 time with your supervisor (start with 5 min). • Work diligently to show appreciation for the work they do, be a good listener.
• Did you have an understanding about email/phone messages on the front end?	• Ask a relevant question in the 1:1 meeting.
• Have you followed up with written requests?	• "Give honest and sincere appreciation" for the answer or discussion.
• Are you using your Dale Carnegie techniques?	• Ask how to improve phone communication going forward.

Dealing With Your Clinical Director

Who Is Constantly Increasing Your Caseload or Offering a Bonus for Increased Billable Hours

The job of the clinical director is a very difficult one; they must oversee the screening and admission of new clients, oversee the work of the BCBAs, and in many cases also manage the clinical budget among other responsibilities. In some companies it may seem like the only job of the clinical director is to crack the whip on billable hours assigned to each behavior analyst. While there may be some of that from a business perspective you also need to consider a few other variables that the clinical director has to deal with. If you are beginning to feel burned out, reflect on the following:

Ask Yourself . . .	***What to Do***
• Have you assessed your current workload, i.e., conducted a time study?	• If not, do this ASAP, use 15-min intervals and put this in a spreadsheet so the clinical director can see how you spend your time.

Ask Yourself . . .	*What to Do*
• Do you have data on client progress?	• Determine if your clients are currently all showing progress on goals, present this graphically.
• Are you able to complete all the necessary supervision time?	• Gather data on your observations of supervisees, trainees, and RBTs, put in a bar graph.
• Was your caseload agreed upon in your job interview?	• Review your interview notes and contract, your clinical director may just be holding you to your agreed upon work assignment.
• Are you starting to feel burned out?	• Do you drag yourself to work, have trouble getting started, disillusioned about your job? Be prepared to push back, do not accept any more cases, are you prepared to give 30-days' notice?

Dealing With Peers and Colleagues (ABA, Non-ABA, Teachers)

Constant Negativity, Lack of Cooperation, Pushing Non-Evidence-Based Procedures

While in graduate school, it is not likely that you will have to deal with a lot of negativity since you are protected by faculty and site supervisors who manage your cases. However, when you take your first job, you will not have much control over the clients with whom you work or the settings where you are assigned. Consider the following questions that you can ask yourself and some suggested responses.

> *If you believe that you are constantly surrounded by difficult people, there is always some chance your demeanor could be a part of the problem.*

Ask Yourself . . .	***What to Do***
• Are you using your Dale Carnegie skills daily with colleagues?	• Review the seven key skills.
• Are you accidentally reinforcing the negativity by engaging with them?	• Remember, arguing is a form of reinforcement.
• Are you shaping on ideas that are a little closer to behavioral treatments?	• Make a concerted effort to listen carefully and reinforce anything constructive.
• Are you educating about advantages of ABA?	• Bring articles to distribute showing clear effects of ABA.

Could You Be the Difficult Person?

People Don't Listen to You, Don't Follow Your Instructions, Are Not Self-motivated

If you believe that you are constantly surrounded by difficult people, there is always some chance your demeanor could be a part of the problem.

If you find that people don't listen to you or follow your directions, you should ask if perhaps you need a different strategy in your interactions with others. The following are some questions you can ask yourself and some suggestions for self-improvement.

Ask Yourself . . .	**What to Do**
• Are you assuming people know what you want from them?	• Break your requirements into smaller segments (use task analysis).
• Do you move too fast with projects?	• Slow down and make sure your supervisees & colleagues can follow your lead.
• Do you expect too much?	• Be more realistic with your expectations.
• Are you too busy to stop and listen?	• Work on your time management (delegate some tasks, keep a daily To-Do list, work on your listening skills).
• Are you stingy with your reinforcers?	• Work on giving more reinforcers more often.

YOUNG PROFESSIONAL (3–5 YEARS)

With a few years' experience in analyzing and managing difficult behaviors, your life should be a little calmer and you should feel like you are not as frazzled at the end of the day. Managing your time and your daily calendar and keeping your priorities clear should result in a manageable workday and supervisees and colleagues who appreciate your work and respect your opinions. With this well-tuned repertoire, it is time to do some mentoring of new BCBAs in your organization to teach them how to analyze the behavior of those around them as well as take stock of their own repertoire. As a seasoned behavior analyst, you will be able to put their frustrations in perspective and offer concrete suggestions on how to get through the day without wanting to just give up and quit.

MID-CAREER (6–10 YEARS)

At this point in your career, you will likely be in at least a junior-management position where you can have some influence on the company's policies and may be able to suggest ways of improving interactions between supervisees, supervisors, BCBAs, and upper management. When the RBTs are saying, "My supervisor doesn't give me enough feedback," or the BCBAs says, "The clinical director is all about accepting new clients and we don't have the staff to provide treatment," consider initiating round-table discussions of common irritations within the company and seeking common solutions. The solutions might involve starting with improved communications and analyzing the contingencies that cause people to be at odds with each other.

SENIOR BEHAVIOR ANALYST

Behavior analysts who have reached senior status have a broad perspective of causal variables that can set the occasion for difficult behaviors. They may have taught courses or workshops on Skinner's Verbal Behavior and have had an opportunity to observe the effects of company-wide contingencies that may have caused problematic behaviors. For example, too great an emphasis on revenue can drive employees to lose track of their fundamental responsibility for their clients' welfare. An inappropriate emphasis on billable hours can pit clinical directors against BCBAs and RBTs. Both BCBAs and RBTs can be pitted against their supervisors, thus increasing unfounded accusations and internal feuding. None of this should occur in a well-run behavior-analytic organization that is led from the top by a leader who understands that there are no difficult people only difficult *behaviors* that have not yet been analyzed and solutions implemented.

SUMMARY

This chapter describes how a behavior analyst would approach the problem of managing difficult people in the workplace. We conceptualize this as difficult *behavior.* A very high percentage of difficult behavior is verbal behavior. This verbal behavior can be analyzed in terms of the speaker-listener relationship where the difficult behavior is maintained by a listener. Further, we describe the analysis of difficult behavior in the context of Friman's *Circumstances View,* i.e., behavior is determined by the immediate environment to a great extent. As behavior analysts, we need to be cognizant of this important variable. To manage difficult behaviors, we assume that behavior analysts can apply what they know about behavior change in general, are willing to apply the principles in the workplace and that they have a basic understanding of Carnegie's classic work, *How to Win Friends and Influence People.*

NOTE

1 Which states that *circumstances* are the cause of problem behavior.

FOR FURTHER READING

Brinkman, R., & Kirschner, R. (2012). *Dealing with people you can't stand: How to bring out the best in people at their worst*. New York: McGraw Hill.

Carnegie, D. C. (2011). *How to win friends and influence people in the digital age*. New York: Simon & Schuster Paperbacks.

Falcone, P. (2019). *101 tough conversations to have with employees* (2nd ed.). New York: Harper Collins.

Tawwab, N. G. (2021). *Set boundaries, find peace: A guide to reclaiming yourself*. New York: Penguin Random House.

Young, D. (2021). *How to deal with difficult people*. Sheridan, WY: GTM Press.

REFERENCES

Carnegie, D. (1981). *How to win friends & influence people*. New York: Gallery Books.

Friman, P. (2021). The circumstances view of problem behavior. *Journal of Applied Behavior Analysis, 54*, 636–653.

Michael, J. (2004). *Concepts and principles of behavior analysis* (rev. ed.). Kalamazoo, MI: Society for the Advancement of Behavior Analysis.

Skinner, B. F. (1957). *Verbal behavior*. Englewood Cliffs, NJ: Prentice-Hall, Inc.

12

Use Shaping Effectively

> ***Shaping, Shaping, Always Shaping.***
>
> **—The tagline of a top-selling product of the Florida Association of Behavior Analysis**

PROLOGUE

Out of frustration, a teacher calls on a third-grade student who is frantically waving her hand and quietly but intensely saying, "Me, me, me!"

On a family trip to New York, a dad, after saying that morning, "Okay, I'll take you to the Apple store, but we're not buying anything today," gets out his platinum credit card and gives in to his begging, pleading 9-year-old daughter.

An arborist supervisor, distracted by an important incoming cell call from the owner, notices that her tree-trimming workers have failed, once again (!) to put on their hard hats, but she hurries to her truck to take the call, saying nothing.

> The ubiquitous power of reinforcement, applied in small dribbles and drabs throughout the day, produces the complex scene of human behavior that unfolds before us as behavior analysts.

The third-grade teacher in the case above is confronted with a student who insists every day on being called on as she

DOI: 10.4324/9781003265573-15

urgently waves her arm and hisses, "Me, me, it's my turn. I know the answer. Puh-leeeze!" Dad has a preteen on his hands who is constantly begging for the latest Earbuds, and the owner of Miller's Tree Service has just received a workers' comp claim regarding an employee who sustained a head injury.

In each case, the principles of behavior were operating to increase ever so slightly the likelihood of inappropriate behavior. Along with this increasing probability of occurrence goes an even greater chance of reinforcement in an ever-increasing circle of settings. The ubiquitous power of reinforcement, applied in small dribbles and drabs throughout the day, produces the complex scene of human behavior that unfolds before us as behavior analysts. Our behavior analytic world is made up of complex, difficult behaviors that require functional analyses to sort out, written behavior plans to change, and formal training protocols, and it often requires patience, tons of patience, to change behaviors. In this sea of accidental reinforcement, behavior analysts are tossed about by waves of inappropriate behavior that will undoubtedly swamp their kayaks if they are not careful. What is a well-trained, conscientious, law-abiding behavior analyst to do?

The laws of behavior operate whether a person is a behavior analyst or not. In each of the three cases above, someone important has engaged in the shaping of inappropriate behavior. The behavioral offenders didn't realize it at the time, and they probably wouldn't admit it if it were pointed out, but just like these seemingly innocuous cases, there are interactions occurring millions of times each day in our culture that add up to a chronic behavioral headache for everyone. These important lessons are usually not explicitly covered in graduate school, and you may not have an opportunity to really use them until you take your first job.

> Our behavior analyst is calm and in charge. She has no reason to get mad or argue with anyone because she knows the observed behavior is the product of the person's reinforcement history, probably going back to childhood.

FRESH OUT OF GRAD SCHOOL, FIRST JOB

Ethics of Shaping

In the hands of a well-trained BCBA fresh out of grad school who has excellent professional skills, shaping can be a joy to behold. Consider the behavior analyst who is in a group of people that includes a very difficult person (Chapter 11). The behavior analyst engages in conversation easily, smiling and nodding her head frequently in conversation. A trained observer might notice that she will occasionally pause, show a neutral expression on her face, and then become engaged again. Amazingly, the stable, popular behavior analyst can make instant calculations as to the likelihood that the behavior she is witnessing is going to eventually cause some trouble. She will apply the smiles, agreements, and head nods at precisely the right time to shape on the behavior of the "difficult person." Our behavior analyst is calm and in charge. She has no reason to get mad or argue with anyone because she knows the observed behavior is the product of the person's reinforcement history, probably going back to childhood.

> Shaping is done accidentally by the untrained and deliberately by the well-trained.

People who could be described as the complainer, the know-it-all, and the drama queen (Bloch, 2005) all present difficulties for everyone around them except the well-grounded behavior analyst, who understands how behavior works. There is a Zen essence to this deep knowledge that gives the behavior analyst not only the calmness that comes with understanding the actions of others, but also the permission to act as needed. Shaping is done accidentally by the untrained and deliberately by the well-trained. Although using behavior analysis in their daily lives is not a requirement, it certainly should not be surprising to discover that individually, behavior analysts can put their knowledge to good use to create some improved degree of appropriate behavior in their realm of influence. Applying what you know about the basic principles of behavior to the people around is in the best interest of you and them.

Everyday Behavior Shaping

In addition to using shaping with clients, you will probably find yourself faced with numerous opportunities every day to use shaping with your supervisor, colleagues, and family members (Sutherland, 2008). Is it ethical to begin using what you learned in school with the people in your daily life? With just a few qualifications, the answer is *yes*. The effect of reinforcement, in the right hands, can be truly powerful. If you hold a reinforcer for a person, know how to use conditioned reinforcers, and are good at your timing, you can deliberately shape some amazing behaviors. But you need to think through a few issues first. You cannot use this knowledge, this deep understanding of human behavior, to promote your own personal agenda. It's not fair, ethical, or appropriate to differentially reinforce your friends for buying you a beer, washing your car, or walking your dog. It's just not right. If you are going to use shaping with the people around you, you must always be ethical about it by selecting behaviors that are in *their* best interests.

For example, suppose you strike up a friendship with someone and discover you have a lot in common, you get along well, and you enjoy spending time together. But this person has an annoying habit of interrupting. It's not malicious, it's not a deal breaker, but you wouldn't want to get caught in an elevator over a weekend with this person, because the constant interrupting would drive you crazy. What should you do? You don't have to bring this annoying habit to the person's attention. Most likely it wouldn't do any good, and in fact, calling attention to the problem could set you back. Shaping is the answer.

> Making shaping look natural so that no one accuses you of being manipulative is a requirement, not an option, for behavior analysts.

Making shaping look natural so that no one accuses you of being manipulative is a requirement, not an option, for behavior analysts. You will lose friends in a hurry if they think you are attempting to trick them into doing something. Your goals must be honorable, and justifiable, not self-serving or demeaning. Sutherland (2008), in her excellent book *What Shamu Taught Me About Life, Love, and Marriage*, described using social reinforcers for all the people around her, from the impatient person in line behind her to her mother who needed to quit smoking and her husband who constantly lost his keys. Sutherland had no qualms about her strategy and was willing to go public with her plans. The media response to her book was overwhelmingly positive. It seemed that most people were enthralled with the idea that one could use the same behavioral procedures used to train animals to improve relationships. In one particularly telling example, Sutherland described how, prior to her use of shaping at home, she enabled her husband's frequently losing his keys by sympathizing with his plight and joining in the frantic search. When she realized what she was doing, let him solve his own problem, and simply reinforced him when he found the keys, the losing became less frequent, and the frenzied searches became calmer and more systematic.

You will be a far more effective behavior analyst if you can develop the habit of looking for behaviors to reinforce wherever you go. At work, you may have colleagues with annoying habits such as borrowing your stapler and not returning it or coming to meetings late. Many people don't feel comfortable giving direct feedback and they let the annoying habits of others simmer until they can't stand it anymore and then explode. Saying, "That's okay," is not a good consequence for someone who has done or said something inconsiderate. Rather, a systematic, consistent plan to *reinforce considerate, responsible behavior* is in order. Sometimes this will clearly rely on the use of shaping, and other times it may not involve successive approximations. If you are a supervisor, feedback and possible documentation (e.g., for a behavior such as tardiness) may be a part of the plan. Note that when we say, "annoying habits," we are not talking about behaviors such as telling inappropriate jokes (e.g., racist, sexist, etc.) which should absolutely not be tolerated, and the appropriate consequence is immediately reporting the person to HR (Human Resources).

Mediators (e.g., teachers and parents who will be carrying out behavioral treatment plans with a child) are particularly sensitive and responsive to well-calculated shaping. They are trying hard and want to please. In their new role as change agents, they may be desperate to know if they are doing what is expected. They are a long way from actually changing a behavior and encountering the natural consequences of their new strategy. The best form of shaping is that which is delivered concurrently with their attempts. Let's look at the situation where the mediator is the mother of an autistic child. You've been trying to teach her to conduct language sessions with the child. You'll want to position yourself so you can observe the interaction between the mother and the child so you can do the shaping that is needed. Sit or stand so the mother can see your face and easily make eye contact. Mom will be able to see your head nod as you encourage training attempts. When she glances your way, a big smile and silently mouthed "Terrific!" or "Great!" will have the desired effect. At the end of the session, you can follow up with immediate, descriptive feedback to show the mother how pleased you are with her progress. You'll be not only increasing the rate of correct responding but also building the confidence and self-assurance that will be needed in the upcoming days when Mom hits a rough patch, and you are not there.

YOUNG PROFESSIONAL (3–5 YEARS)

Develop the Shaping Habit

After your first couple of years in your new job, you may become more aware of opportunities to shape on the behavior of people around you. Supervisees need to become more independent and not rely on daily feedback, your BCaBA needs to pick up the slack in providing supervision, and a colleague that you befriended is starting to take up too much time with personal issues. All of these problems can be tackled by careful shaping.

Behavior analysts interact with dozens or even hundreds of people each week so the opportunities for shaping are enormous, but, as with most acquisition tasks, it is probably best to start small. In the beginning, you will need to select one or two people and one or two behaviors for each person. With shaping, you are not trying to produce a totally new behavior but rather aiming to increase the probability that some particular response will occur more often or at the right time. Exercising your shaping skills during a discussion with colleagues or an important meeting with administrators presents a different sort of opportunity.

MID-CAREER (6–10 YEARS)

Once you reach mid-career status, behavior shaping should be automatic, intuitive, and a smooth and seamless part of your repertoire. This skill can be used to run meetings efficiently, energize your board of directors, cool down your overly aggressive PR firm, and tame your new employees who may be a little too eager to rock the boat. As an administrator yourself, you will see the power of shaping to influence the decisions your C-suite colleagues need to make on a weekly basis. Depending on your position and time in grade, your skill in shaping will help you influence the direction that your company takes and the influence it has on the community.

SENIOR BEHAVIOR ANALYST

After a decade in the field and with hundreds of successful shaping projects under your belt, you should be able to take charge of your company and apply your techniques on a broader scale. You may run into people from other provider companies, funding organizations, government agencies, or legislative committees whom you could bring around to be more willing to listen, more cooperative, and perhaps more amenable to your ideas. Shaping involves the delivery of reinforcers in a tactical manner so that you get two-for-one: the reinforcement itself provides a pairing with you so that people will find you more interesting to be around, and if you can work your magic with the shaping contingency, you should see slight changes in behavior. Everyone likes a person who delivers reinforcers. Being a reinforcing person will get you into the room, and once there, shaping is essential to grease the wheels of agreement and harmony.

SUMMARY

Chapter 12: Use Shaping Effectively

"Shaping, Shaping, Always Shaping." This mantra repeated slowly and occasionally throughout the day with your voice pitched an octave lower than normal serves as a reminder that you, as the behavior analyst consultant, *can* influence the behavior of people around you. This chapter describes how behavior analysts can use shaping in their work settings. It is entirely ethical to use shaping in the best interest of others to improve their performance, reduce their irritating or aversive behavior, or improve their appropriate behavior and productivity. Using shaping simply to benefit the person who is doing the shaping is not ethical. Becoming practiced at shaping means looking for opportunities everywhere to reinforce interesting, effective, and pro-social behaviors.

FOR FURTHER READING

Friman, P. (2021). The circumstances view of problem behavior. *Journal of Applied Behavior Analysis*, *54*, 636–653.

REFERENCES

Bloch, J. P. (2005). *Handling difficult people.* Avon, MA: Adams Media.

Sutherland, A. (2008). *What Shamu taught me about life, love, and marriage.* New York: Random House.

13

Diversity, Equity, and Inclusion

When you know better, you do better.
—Maya Angelou[1]

FIRST SOME BACKGROUND

In addition to being competent in the technical aspects of their jobs, behavior analysts should also be decent people who treat others fairly and make everyone feel welcome and respected. Demonstrating the importance of how behavior analysts treat others, in the BACB's Code of Ethics (Behavior Analysis Certification Board, 2020) that became effective on January 1, 2022, there were some new items that stressed the importance of critical concepts such as diversity, equity, inclusion, and cultural responsiveness.

While Diversity, Equity, and Inclusion (DEI) training is just appearing in the 2020 Code, there has been training on these topics in corporate settings since the 1960s (Lussier, 2020). In the mid-1960s, equal employment law and affirmative action called attention to employment issues that were based on race and there was a call for change.

Of the four core principles in the Code that all behavior analysts should follow, two relate to equity and cultural responsiveness. Core Principle #2 is to *Treat Others with Compassion, Dignity, and Respect.*

DOI: 10.4324/9781003265573-16

Specifically, the Code says that:

> behavior analysts are to treat others equitably, regardless of factors such as age, disability, ethnicity, gender expression/identity, immigration status, marital/relationship status, national origin, race, religion, sexual orientation, socioeconomic status, or any other basis proscribed by law.

Related to this, Core Principle #4 is that behavior analysts will *Ensure their Competence.* "Behavior analysts ensure their competence by working to continually increase their knowledge and skills related to cultural responsiveness and service delivery to diverse groups."

In addition to Core Principles related to diversity, equity, inclusion, and cultural responsiveness, specific Code items (1.07, 1.08, 1.10, and 4.07) are now included on these important topics.

CULTURAL RESPONSIVENESS

Cultural responsiveness (see Chapter 9) for behavior analysts means that in addition to being aware of one's own culture, the behavior analyst will be aware of, and will learn about, the cultural and community norms of the clients and families they serve. Clients and families who are minorities should be supported (Khalifa, Gooden, & Davis, 2016) and their cultural views should be considered when planning and delivering services. Cultural Responsiveness basically means being responsive to the culture of someone different than you. The need for behavior analysis professionals to incorporate culturally responsive practices is especially important considering the projected increase in diversity in the United States (Beaulieu & Jimenez-Gomez, 2022).

> Cultural Humility means reflecting on yourself, while Cultural Responsiveness means that you reflect on and consider the cultures of others.

CULTURAL HUMILITY

Closely related to cultural responsiveness is *Cultural Humility.* Introduced in 1998 by the physical healthcare field, the term

Cultural Humility is the lifelong process focusing on self-reflection and personal critique and acknowledging one's biases (Khan, 2021). A key characteristic of cultural humility is that the therapist will work towards reducing the power imbalance between the client/family and therapist, and the therapist will not adopt an attitude of superiority. In the big picture, Cultural Humility means reflecting on yourself, while Cultural Responsiveness means that you reflect on and consider the cultures of others.

CULTURAL COMPETENCE

There are many definitions of cultural competence, and this term has received increased attention in recent years in professions such as medicine, counseling, social work, and psychology (Sue, Sue, Neville, & Smith, 2019). As with cultural humility, cultural competence is a lifelong process during which one works to create conditions that will maximize the optimal development of the client (Sue & Torino, 2005). Cultural competence means that behavior analysts will be equally responsive to all groups of clients, and they will communicate and intervene on behalf of all of their clients. To become culturally competent, behavior analysts must be sensitive to the cultural practices of others.

Finally, once you begin to reflect on yourself (regarding biases) and the cultural and community norms of others, it is time to put these reflections into action. This is done by adopting practices related to Diversity, Equity, and Inclusion.

FRESH OUT OF GRAD SCHOOL, FIRST JOB

As soon as you begin your first job, in addition to technical training on behavior analytic skills, it is important for you to receive training and be aware of the concepts of diversity, equity, and inclusion that are described subsequently. This is the time for you to begin reflecting on whether you have biases and if you do, how you can respond to address these biases. At this stage in your career, you are not likely to be able to control policy, but you can work on yourself, speak up in meetings or DEI training, and you can report any instances you see that relate to discrimination or biases.

Diversity

Diversity means including people from a different range of social and ethnic backgrounds, ages, genders or sexual orientations, religions, national origins, and so on.

Years ago, diversity in the workplace was mostly focused on race, gender, and age. In more recent years, the diversity conversation also includes physical ability, ethnicity, sexual orientation, religion, and other factors such as education, work experience, parental status, immigration status, income, and relationship status.

> Tina moved from an urban area to a smaller city and accepted a job at a behavioral consulting firm. The company was started several years ago by Heather, a BCBA-D. When Heather left a larger company and went out on her own, in the beginning, she was the only consultant. Before long, she hired a behavioral acquaintance, Megan. And soon after that, she hired additional consultants that she felt would "fit in nicely with the group." Tina soon realized the new company had no diversity. All the BCBAs were 26 to 40-year-old millennials. They were all Caucasian, and they were all female. Maybe Heather was a racist, maybe not. It could have been that no one else applied for the jobs, or Heather just got in the habit of hiring people who were like herself. One thing is for sure—this is not a diverse workplace.

It is our job as behavior analysis professionals to protect the clients that we serve. In addition to advocating quality services, behavior analysts should be aware of biased and discriminatory practices in our field. Currently, Black children experience racial disparities regarding the timing of the diagnosis of ASD (autism spectrum disorder) and they may be more likely to be incorrectly classified with intellectual disabilities (Constantino et al., 2020).

Because Latino and Black children are less likely to be diagnosed with ADHD (Coker et al., 2016), behavior analysts should pay close attention to make sure all children are getting the services they deserve.

Equity

Equity basically means being just, fair, and impartial, and it relates to providing everyone with what they need to succeed.

Equity implies a willingness to make adjustments to ensure others succeed. As an example, with behavior analysis clients, equity could mean that you identify problems that a client is having (e.g., Amari is having a difficult time learning to read), then you provide adequate resources for learning (such as access to a computer the family cannot afford) and provide the support the family needs to help their child. These steps create an equitable situation for a family with limited financial resources.

The basic idea behind inclusion is to help everyone feel welcome and accepted.

You may also hear the term *equality*. Both equity and equality are terms typically related to racial justice. Equality means that everyone is treated the same way. In a behavior analysis company, all employees should have the same opportunities for raises, additional benefits, to make progress in their careers, and so on. There should be no discrimination based on characteristics such as physical ability, ethnicity, sexual orientation, religion, and other factors such as education, work experience, parental status, immigration status, income, and relationship status.

It is possible to have equality without equity. There is a saying in the social change literature by an unknown author that says, "Equality is giving everyone the same pair of shoes. Equity is giving everyone a pair of shoes that fits" (Risetowin.org, 2022).

Inclusion

Inclusion means including everyone, no matter their age, disability, ethnicity, gender expression/identity, immigration status, marital/relationship status, national origin, race, religion, sexual orientation, or socioeconomic status. The basic idea behind inclusion is to help everyone feel welcome and accepted.

> Jen and Sara were behavior analysts who worked at a large consulting firm. On a Wednesday morning, they both went into the breakroom to get coffee. Roger, another employee, was seated at

a table nearby. Jen said to Sara, "Wasn't that hysterical last night when Tim started doing those impressions of movie stars. I couldn't stop laughing . . ." Roger spoke up and asked, "What are you talking about?" Jen said, "We all went out for Taco Tuesday. Tim was doing impressions to entertain us." With a sad look, Roger said, "That sounds like fun. I wish I had been invited." Squirming and avoiding eye contact, Sara looked at her watch and said she need to get back to her desk. Jen told Roger, "Roger, I am so sorry. I was the person who did the inviting. I just didn't think you would be comfortable going to that place since you are in a wheelchair and there are stairs in the front."

This was a sad situation. If Jen had gone out with one or two friends, that would have been fine. But in this case, everyone in the department was invited except Roger. This was certainly not an example of inclusion. Roger could have been invited, and Jen could have privately mentioned to him that accessibility might be a problem. She could have offered to call the restaurant and ask about parking and an elevator. Or, she could have asked Roger if he would prefer to call the restaurant.

Inclusion in the case above would have meant 1) inviting everyone, 2) giving Roger a choice as to how to handle the accessibility issue, or 3) finding another place that was wheelchair accessible where everyone, including Roger, would feel comfortable.

Code standard 1.08, Nondiscrimination, overlaps somewhat with other Code items related to equity and inclusion. Code 1.08 says that behavior analysts do not discriminate against others. With very few exceptions, we believe that behavior analysts explicitly discriminating against others is not a large or frequent problem. The real problem relates to the discrimination of behavior analysts by others.

Mariana was a Latina behavior analyst who was discriminated against because of her accent. While she was very bright, hardworking, extremely qualified, and a top-notch clinician, Mariana was not considered for a behavior analysis consulting position because she was perceived, unfairly, by the company owner to be less competent than some of the other consultants. In this case, the discrimination involved a company that was hiring. The company owner was not a behavior analyst so no action could be taken against him by the Board, but Mariana could certainly file a discrimination claim with her state administrative agency or the Equal Employment Opportunity Commission (EEOC).

While some discrimination against behavior analysts involves an agency, other times, it is the family or client that is engaging in discrimination. Darrel was a male BCBA who worked for months with a child in the home. Darrel got great reviews from the child's parents. On one Friday visit, the autumn weather had turned crisp and cool—it was just perfect. The mother asked Darrel how he would spend the weekend. "Oh, you're going hiking . . . will you go with your girlfriend or wife?" she said. Not wanting to lie, Darrel replied, "Well, I am married, but I'm married to a man." Within 24 hours, the mother called the company and demanded another consultant. This was a clear case of discrimination against a behavior analyst based on sexual orientation.

Unfortunately, but understandably, the Code only pertains to behavior analysts. In the cases above, if the owner of the company who chose to not hire the Latina behavior analyst was not a behavior analyst, the person does not come under the Code. If the parent who discriminated against the male behavior analyst who disclosed he was married to a man was not a behavior analyst, that parent does not come under the Code either. We all need to work together to determine how best to handle situations in which our behavior analysts are not receiving the respect that they so richly deserve and educate everyone about how to handle discrimination cases beyond the BACB.

Levels of Bias

Code standard 1.10 refers to the personal biases of behavior analysts. A somewhat controversial trend in current DEI training across multiple fields is teaching that everyone has biases. Unfortunately, this is often interpreted as everyone, deep down inside, has racist, sexist, or other truly unacceptable, offensive biases. There are different levels of bias.

1. General Unawareness

This is self-explanatory. It means that sometimes there is a bias because the person is just not aware of the issue. While it certainly should be corrected, it is often innocent.

> Rodney and Becca, two enthusiastic behavior analysts at a large consulting firm, were asked by a director to work together to plan a weekend day with a bonding activity for all staff. In the past, the company had picnics and had gone bowling, but the director said she wanted more, and she wanted the activity to require everyone to participate. Rodney and Becca decided on having everyone attend a "Ropes" course where staff would be assigned to competitive teams and would need to climb, walk on swinging bridges, zipline, and climb across nets. This activity was ultimately vetoed by another director, who realized that some staff had physical issues that would prevent them from being successful. The two 20-something-year-olds were simply unaware, and once they heard the explanation, they became more sensitive.

2. Lack of Knowledge

In general, people are getting to be more knowledgeable, but there are still some situations in which people have a bias that is due to a lack of knowledge. This can apply when a behavior analyst goes into the home of a family from a different culture, country, or religion and does not understand their preferences.

> Bill was a BCBA who was assigned to start working with a client in the home. There was an initial intake session, but apparently, it was not complete enough. Bill was getting frustrated and telling his supervisor, "This mom is a pain. I don't think she really wants these services. I text her and ask if I can come at a certain time and she always says 'no.' We have other clients to see. This mom is not cooperating."
>
> Somehow, Bill was operating without critical information, and he had a lack of knowledge about this family's culture and religion. The family was Muslim. They prayed a certain number of times during the day and their schedule had to accommodate this. Further, the mom was not to be alone with a man. The case manager, a female, finally talked to the mother, got the necessary

information, and developed a plan that was appropriate for the family. Bill was assigned to another case and a female behavior analyst replaced him.

3. *Implicit (Unconscious) Bias*

With implicit bias, there is usually a preference for (or aversion to) a group of people. Stereotypes are often associated with the group. Examples would be, "This (specified) group of people would be more likely to mug you when you are walking down the street," or "High school students from this (specified) country are more likely to do better at math."

Mary was a 60-something-year-old professional woman. Late one afternoon, she decided to go alone to dinner at a local steak restaurant. The restaurant was an informal place with wooden booths and the guests threw peanut shells on the floor. When Mary arrived, due to the early hour, there were only two couples in the restaurant. The hostess greeted Mary and led her to a table at the very back of the restaurant. It was around a corner and faced the open door of the kitchen. "Could I have another table—like in the restaurant part," said Mary. The hostess (who happened to be a young woman) said, "No, this is all we've got." "I don't get it," Mary replied, "There is no one here and there are plenty of tables." The hostess refused to seat Mary (who was still standing) at another table. Mary left and went 1-mile down the road to an Outback Steakhouse. She walked in and was greeted by a hostess who said, "Welcome to Outback. It's early. We're wide open—where would you like to sit?"

There is a lot more to this story that involved Mary writing to the district manager about the first restaurant. But what is relevant here is how biases are developed from a learning history. Anyone who has waited tables will tell you that women are thought of as notoriously bad tippers. They are often asked if they want to sit at the bar or near the noisy kitchen (rather than take up a nice table). The hostess could have had this "bad tipper" bias. And Mary could have developed a bias related to younger people because of the way she was treated. This case involved both the hostess's bias against women and perhaps women of a certain age group, and the possible development of a bias Mary would come to have toward younger restaurant workers.

> Related to behavior analysis and age issues, if a behavior analyst is young, clients/families may think they lack the necessary experience. If the behavior analyst is older, there could be a bias related to the family thinking the behavior analyst is not current with research and modern techniques.

It is important to understand when reflecting on one's own biases that behavior can represent what is true about some members of a group, but not all.

4. Explicit (Conscious) Bias

Explicit bias is what is traditionally thought of as *bias*. With explicit bias, individuals are aware of their attitudes and any prejudice they have toward a specific group. Explicit biases are conscious. Examples of explicit bias are racist comments or comments/behavior toward any other marginalized group.

> Sadly, one of the most frequent examples of explicit bias involves discriminating against someone based on their race. White families will sometimes ask to have a behavior analyst who is "more like us" if they are assigned a Black behavior analyst. Companies will have to decide if they want to work with clients who exhibit explicit biases.
>
> One possible way to handle this is to include statements on the company's web page and Service Agreement that spells out before services even begin, "We strive to be a diverse company and we are proud of all of our consultants. We do not tolerate discrimination based on age, disability, ethnicity, gender expression/identity, immigration status, marital/relationship status, national origin, race, religion, sexual orientation, or socioeconomic status. Our consultants are well-trained, highly skilled, and senior consultants are certified through the Behavior Analysis Certification Board."

Code standard 4.07 refers to the need for supervisors to train supervisees and trainees on topics related to diversity (e.g., age, disability, ethnicity, gender expression/identity, immigration status, marital/relationship status, national origin, race, religion, sexual orientation, and socioeconomic status). Supervisors must also incorporate the training into the behavior analyst's work.

Benefits to Diversity

There are many benefits to diversity. These can include increased creativity, innovation, higher employee engagement/retention, more career opportunities, increased revenue and financial performance, and better marketing opportunities. Diversity, when paired with inclusion and equity, leads to extraordinary results.

YOUNG PROFESSIONAL (3–5 YEARS)

By now you have had DEI training and you have reflected on any biases you might have. You may have begun to work in diverse treatment settings with people who differ from you regarding race, religion, sexual orientation, gender identification, age, religion, disability, and so on. You are in a position to model for new behavior analysts how to work with others as a part of a team. This is a time when you can continue to learn about and appreciate everyone including all your co-workers and the families to whom you provide services and provide a role model for new BCBAs joining the company.

MID-CAREER (6–10 YEARS)

As a mid-career behavior analyst, you are probably supervising others and may be in a leadership position where you can teach supervisees and trainees about DEI and help them examine and address any biases they might have. You can attend DEI training at state and national conferences to learn more about helping others with their biases. You can also interact with your supervisor or company owner about how your agency can improve regarding DEI training, increasing diversity, becoming more equitable, and fostering inclusion.

SENIOR BEHAVIOR ANALYST

As a senior behavior analyst, you are likely to be able to change and make company policy. You might own the company, so that when a parent discriminates against one of your behavior analysts, you can decide how the discrimination will be handled. Think about the previous case of Darrel, who revealed that he was gay, and the family wanted him gone. As a company owner, what do you do? You can decide you will discontinue the services provided to the family, or you can attempt to change the mindset of the parents. You can support Darrel and find him a setting where he can be appreciated. You can sit on committees or organize a committee of local agencies so you can all talk about how to handle issues related to discrimination.

SUMMARY

This chapter addressed diversity, equity, and inclusion as well as related topics such as cultural humility, cultural responsiveness, and cultural competence. Cultural humility involves reflecting on your own biases, whether they are implicit or explicit. Cultural responsiveness for behavior analysts means that behavior analysts should be aware of and learn about the cultural and community norms of the clients and families they serve, and cultural competence means that behavior analysts will communicate and intervene on behalf of all their clients. The Code of Ethics for Behavior Analysts now recognizes as critical for the training and practices of behavior analysts: Cultural Responsiveness and Diversity (1.07), Nondiscrimination (1.08), Awareness of Personal Biases and Challenges (1.10), and Incorporating and Addressing Diversity (4.07). In the future, individual behavior analysts, companies, and our field will need to learn how to best handle situations where someone is not valued or treated with the respect that they deserve.

NOTE

1 www.oprah.com/oprahs-lifeclass/the-powerful-lesson-maya-angelou-taught-oprah-video. There are several versions of this quote on the internet (Winfrey, 2011).

REFERENCES

Beaulieu, L., & Jimenez-Gomez, C. (2022). Cultural responsiveness in applied behavior analysis: Self-assessment. *Journal of Applied Behavior Analysis*, *55*, 337–356.

Behavior Analysis Certification Board. (2020, updated March 2022). *Ethics code for behavior analysts*. Retrieved July 3, 2022, from www.bacb.com/wp-content/uploads/2022/01/Ethics-Code-for-Behavior-Analysts-220316-2.pdf

Coker, T. R., Elliott, M. N., Toomey, S. L., Schwebel, D. C., Cuccaro, P., Emery, S. T., Davies, S. L., Visser, S. N., & Schuster, M. A. (2016). Racial and ethnic disparities in ADHA diagnosis and treatment. *Pediatrics*, *138*(3), e20160407. https://doi.org/10.1542/peds.2016-0407

Constantino, J. N., Abbacchi, A. M., Saulnier, C., Klaiman, C., Mandell, D., Zhang, Y., Hawks, Z., Bates, J., Klin, A., Shattuck, P., Molholm, S., Fitzgerald, R., Roux, A., Loew, J. K., & Geschwind, D. H. (2020). Timing of the diagnosis of autism in African American children. *Pediatrics*, *146*(3), 1–9. https://doi.org/10.1542/peds.2019-3629

Khalifa, M., Gooden, M. A., & Davis, J. E. (2016). Culturally responsive school leadership: A synthesis of the literature. *Review of Educational Research*, *86*(4), 1272–1311.

Khan, S. (2021). Cultural humility vs. cultural competence—Why providers need both. *Health City*. Retrieved July 3, 2022, from https://healthcity.bmc.org/policy-and-industry/cultural-humility-vs-cultural-competence-providers-need-both

Lussier, K. (2020). What the history of diversity training reveals about its future. *The Conversation*. Retrieved July 2, 2022, from https://theconversation.com/what-the-history-of-diversity-training-reveals-about-its-future

Risetowin.org. (2022). *Equality vs. equity*. Retrieved July 17, 2022, from https://risetowin.org/what-we-do/educate/resource-module/equality-vs-equity/index.html#:~:text=Begin%20by%20briefly%20explaining%20the,pair%20of%20shoes%20that%20fits.%E2%80%9D

Sue, D. W., Sue, D., Neville, H. A., & Smith, L. (2019). *Counseling the culturally diverse: Theory and practice*. Hoboken, NJ: John Wiley & Sons.

Sue, D. W., & Torino, G. C. (2005). Racial-cultural competence: Awareness, knowledge, and skills. In R. T. Carter (Ed.), *Handbook of racial-cultural psychology and counseling*. Hoboken, NJ: John Wiley & Sons.

Winfrey, O. (2011, October 19). *Oprah's life class*. Retrieved July 3, 2022, from www.oprah.com/oprahs-lifeclass/the-powerful-lesson-maya-angelou-taught-oprah-video

14

Performance Management

> ***Performance Management is a systematic, data-oriented approach to managing people at work that relies on positive reinforcement as the major way to maximize performance.***
>
> **—Aubrey Daniels**

FRESH OUT OF GRAD SCHOOL, FIRST JOB

As a graduate student, you may not have had a course in Performance Management (PM) or Organizational Behavior Management (OBM),[1] yet on your first job you may be presented with performance issues that are major challenges. RBTs may not have a good work ethic (showing up late or not at all for client sessions, not collecting data reliably, etc.) or the necessary professional skills for dealing with teachers, parents, or stakeholders. When you encounter problems from several staff, it may be necessary to set

> The application of performance management can establish a solid foundation for employee relations, reduced turnover, rapid acquisition of clinical skills, and loyalty to the organization and its mission.

DOI: 10.4324/9781003265573-17

up performance management systems that will effectively train, prompt, and maintain appropriate behaviors for the whole team.

The basic principles of behavior as we know them are no different when implemented directly with an individual client than when they are applied to the staff of an ABA agency or the "associates" at an Amazon fulfilment center. When dealing with the performance of behavior technicians, the targets are different in that they are not clinical problems, that is, you are not dealing with maladaptive, self-injurious, or aggressive behaviors, but rather with unskilled, inefficient, unproductive, unsafe, or costly behaviors. These behaviors, all considered "normal" rather than *clinical* for almost any work environment, are incredibly common, and they cause consternation among supervisors, clinical directors, and CEOs who may resort to termination or aversive control as a management tool. The application of performance management can establish a solid foundation for employee relations, reduced turnover, rapid acquisition of clinical skills, and loyalty to the organization and its mission. If managers of ABA companies ignore the fundamentals of performance management, they will almost certainly see disgruntled employees filing complaints against supervisors or the company, high turnover, and a subsequent loss of clients, revenue, and a tainted reputation in the community. In some cases, serious problems with staff morale and a lack of good management can put an entire organization at risk of losing its funding base. If staff members are not doing their jobs and providing quality programming (and supervisors are not making this happen), the ultimate cost can be significant. In business

Unfortunately, in the last few years, as ABA has become monetized, there has been a rising interest in using performance management to increase caseloads, reduce supervision, enhance production, and boost billable hours regardless of clients' needs for service.

settings, these common behavior and management problems can cost huge sums when scaled across a fiscal year for hundreds or thousands of employees not to mention the untold cost to clients.

Performance Management in Human Services Settings

Performance Management has its roots in business and industry applications (Daniels & Bailey, 2014; Rodriguez, 2021). Unfortunately, in the last few years, as ABA has become monetized, there has been a rising interest in using performance management to increase caseloads, reduce supervision, enhance production, and boost billable hours regardless of clients' needs for service. We do not advocate this approach except in rare circumstances and rather support the goal of improving the *quality* of client services by enhancing the skills of the therapists and other staff (Reid, 1998; Reid, Parsons, & Green, 2012).

First A Referral

Under normal circumstances, a company will seek input from a behavioral consulting firm such as Aubrey Daniels International or ALULA. However, as a new BCBA grad, if you have had a course in PM and have carried out some projects, you may want to take on a project with your team of RBTs, trainees, and BCaBAs. You will essentially be making a referral to yourself.[2] PM in a human services setting might involve issues with RBTs not following the behavior plan or not taking data properly. Or the problem could be BCaBAs are not doing a very good job of supervising their trainees, missing appointments, being vague about feedback, or not keeping good records.

Next Pinpointing

Aubrey Daniels (2000) is credited with starting the field of PM in the mid-1960s; he refers to identifying an actual behavior problem as *pinpointing*, that is, converting a vague reference to a workplace issue into observable, measurable behaviors. "Not following the behavior plan" would need to be operationally defined such that a task analysis could be used by a trained observer. "Not doing a good job of supervising" would require a data checklist of good supervisory behaviors such as starting with a greeting, making eye contact, and praising some appropriate behavior followed by a brief description of the immediate problem to be addressed. This script could be made into an observation form which could then be used to measure the baseline level of supervisory behavior.

Then Measurement

Before embarking on any PM project, it is necessary to measure the problem at hand. It is generally recognized that there are four categories of measurement (Gilbert, 1978): *quality, quantity, timeliness, and cost.* One of the most important measures in behavior analysis is that the quality of services that are delivered is measured primarily by *protocol integrity,* i.e., did the therapist follow the required treatment plan exactly as written (see Chapter 6 for more on this). The second measure has to do with improvement in client behaviors that have been targeted. Here the measures may be of the *quality* of the performance, e.g., language acquisition or social skills, or by *quantity,* e.g., how much a SIB was reduced or the amount of the increase in tasks completed. For an extensive discussion of measurement issues, see Chapter 7 in Daniels & Bailey, 2014. Once you have established the pinpoint and have enough baseline measures to determine if the referred problem is in fact stable and socially significant, the next step is to analyze the pinpoint to see if you can find the functional variables. To do this we recommend using a diagnostic approach based on Mager and Pipe's (1970) troubleshooting algorithm. This algorithm is designed to be used by business managers in industrial settings and it consists of a series of questions designed to help the manager find the cause of a performance discrepancy. Possible causes included in Mager and Pipe's (1970) model included a skill deficiency, i.e., did the person ever receive training on the task? Uncovering obstacles that prevent the person from performing the task and finding ways of simplifying the task were also included. Gilbert (1978) and Kent (1985) espoused a similar strategy that Bailey and Austin (1996) later modified and put into a least-to-most intrusive sequence. Bailey (1998) expanded the questions and adapted them for use in human services environments. Using diagnostic questions in applied settings has been validated in published research (Ditzian, Wilder, King, & Tanz, 2015).

A Dozen Diagnostic Questions (Bailey, 1998)

1. Does the person understand what behavior is expected? Have clear goals and objectives been identified?
2. Does the person actually have the skill? Has it been demonstrated in the past?
3. Is there a specific prompt for the behavior in the setting where the task should occur?
4. Is the person's BCBA providing the required number of hours of supervision? Does it appear to be *effective* supervision? (See Chapter 13 for more on this.)
5. Does the employee have a personal problem preventing the behavior that requires counseling or clinical treatment?
6. If equipment is required, does it work? Is it in good repair?
7. Is the task designed to be carried out in an efficient fashion? Can it be streamlined or eliminated? Is the environment conducive to high performance?
8. Is there any unintended, taxing *response effort* or *response cost* associated with performing the task?
9. Does the behavior produce an observable effect that the person can perceive, e.g., a change in the client's behavior?
10. Is a competing behavior being reinforced, e.g., talking on the phone, checking email and text messages?
11. Does the person receive any positive feedback of any kind (vocal, written, graphic) from clients, stakeholders, supervisors, or the agency for their performance?
12. Is there any intrinsic reinforcement for the behavior? Any tangible extrinsic reinforcement?

Using the Questions to Find Functional Variables

Each question is intended to prompt an inquiry on your part; it also suggests a solution. For example, if for Q. #1 clear goals and objectives have not been specified for the person, you would make sure that this was implemented and documented. For Q. #5, before embarking on any intensive intervention it is a good idea to determine if the trainee or staff person has some financial, personal, emotional, or psychological issue that is troubling them. If so, then a referral to HR would be in order. For Q. #6, if you detect an equipment issue that makes the job of the behavior analyst difficult, e.g., they must collect data with pen and paper since the software they are required to use does not work properly on their iPad, you will want to make sure to get the equipment fixed before setting up any unfair contingencies. If you get all the way to Q. #12 and determine that what you have is a motivation issue, it may be necessary to look at ways of building in some form of intrinsic motivation. If that is not possible, an extrinsic system such as a token or point system to reward the completion of certain onerous tasks is needed. Such systems are complex to set up and maintain so you make sure that you have carefully considered questions 1–11 before embarking on this solution.

Whatever intervention you choose should be implemented with integrity, and it should include respecting the dignity of the staff member.

A Functional Intervention

The Dozen Diagnostic Questions are designed to prompt you to seek interventions that are from least-to-most intrusive, i.e., making clear to an RBT that what is expected as a first step is a low-cost intervention vs. setting up a token or bonus system to motivate the performance. It is expected that as a behavior analyst you will be able to look at your baseline data and determine if an intervention is needed (i.e., the behavior is socially significant, and the data are stable) following standard ABA research guidelines (Bailey & Burch, 2018). Whatever intervention you choose should be implemented with integrity, and it should include respecting the dignity of the staff member.

Evaluation

As a BCBA, you know that all interventions must be evaluated. These evaluations are easily done using single-case designs which are perfect for evaluating an intervention with one person or with several therapists. If you had a stable baseline prior to intervention your next task is to determine if there was an effect and if the effect was socially significant. Since the questions are arranged in descending order according to intrusiveness and/or complexity/cost, going to the next level means you need to be ready to engage in more effort to try and correct the problem. As shown in Figure 14.1, a series of interventions were required to improve the quality of the training delivered to the client. Quality was at zero for the initial observations. After goals were clarified there was no improvement, prompts were added that had no effect, and when training was implemented, there was a small improvement. The functional variable that had the greatest effect was adding effective supervision on top of the training.

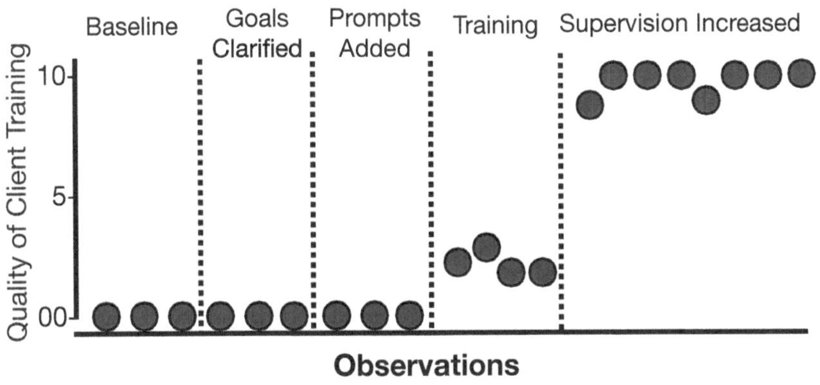

Figure 14.1 This figure shows how the BCBA tested several hypotheses with regard to a therapist's performance with clients. It seems clear from this hypothetical data that clarifying goals and adding prompts had no effect. It was only after training followed by improved supervision that the quality improved.

YOUNG PROFESSIONAL (3–5 YEARS)

As you become more practiced in the use of the diagnostic questions with your RBTs and BCaBAs, you will likely be able to prevent performance problems in your unit. Knowing ahead of time that you need to make goals clear to all your staff and that they should be properly trained for each task (most likely using BST) means that you will have fewer problems in the future. You will be able to train your BCaBAs to use the Diagnostic Questions as well as make them more effective as trainers and supervisors.

MID-CAREER (6–10 YEARS)

When you reach this level as a professional, you should be in a position as an administrator to employ the general methods of Performance Management and institute the diagnostic questions model throughout the organization to solve larger problems that may be chronic in nature. Turnover, for example, needs to be closely studied to determine variables that are operative. Simply paying people more may not be enough to change performance, although this is often the first thing tried by organizations that are having problems. Arranging exit interviews with departing staff and professionals is frequently recommended by HR departments. This approach assumes that people feel comfortable talking about their reasons for leaving. Some reasons that a person leaves a company may be out of control of the company, such as the employee is moving because the spouse or partner got a job in another state. Unfortunately, some of the reasons a person leaves may be uncomfortable to hear. These reasons could relate to how they have been treated or not supported by supervisors, how they believe that there is unethical conduct at the top of the organization, or they have persistent concerns about nepotism or multiple relationships ingrained in the company. These sorts of organizational failures will require a different set of diagnostic questions aimed at the ethical fabric of the whole company.

SENIOR BEHAVIOR ANALYST

With over a decade in the field and perhaps at the same company where you started years ago, you will likely now be in a position to take a broad view of the field of behavior analysis and your organization. You will be able to draw big conclusions about how your company should be reorganized to optimize human performance using all the tools of Performance Management and the basic concepts behind the diagnostic questions. Goals should be set for all members of the treatment team; appropriate prompts should be included in the work environment and all associates from therapists to clinical directors should receive appropriate training so that all the skills they need are at hand. It goes without saying that a critical form of support is that the hardware and software is in good repair and the work environment is safe and hazard-free.

Finally, it seems so logical, but any task that employees are expected to complete should involve some kind of observable outcome that can serve as a form of automatic feedback and reinforcement.

SUMMARY

This chapter described the field of Performance Management. Performance Management (PM) is derived from the basic principles of behavior that have been developed over the past 50 years to improve human performance in business and industry. Adapted for use in human service settings, PM uses diagnostic questions and procedures such as conducting a functional analysis to improve the performance of trainees, staff, and other personnel.

NOTES

1 There is a professional organization that you can join called The Organizational Behavior Management Network. Here is a link to their website: **http://obmnetwork.com**

2 You will, of course, want to consult with your clinical director first to make sure that there are no objections.

FOR FURTHER READING

Abernathy, W. B. (2011). *Pay for profit: Designing an organization-wide performance-based compensation system*. Memphis: PerfSys Press.

Abernathy, W. B. (2014). *The liberated workplace: Transitioning to walden three*. Atlanta, GA: Performance Management Publications.

Austin, J., & Carr, J. E. (2000). *Handbook of applied behavior analysis*. Reno, NV: Context Press.

Bailey, J. S., & Burch, M. R. (2022). *How to think like a behavior analyst* (2nd ed.). New York: Routledge, Inc.

Brethower, D. M. (1972). *Behavior analysis in business and industry: A total performance system*. Kalamazoo, MI: Behaviordelia, Inc.

Daniels, A. C. (2009). *Oops! 13 Management practices that waste time and money (and what to do instead)*. Atlanta, GA: Performance Management Publications.

Daniels, A., C., & Daniels, J. E. (2005). *Measure of a leader: An actionable formula for legendary leadership*. Atlanta, GA: Performance Management Publications.

Gawande, A. (2009). *The checklist manifesto: How to get things done right*. New York, NY: Metropolitan Books.

Iwata, B. A., Smith, R. G., & Michael, J. (2000). Current research on the influence of establishing operations on behavior in applied settings. *Journal of Applied Behavior Analysis*, *33*(4), 411–418.

Komaki, J. (1998). *Leadership from an operant perspective*. New York, NY: Routledge.

Mager, R. F., & Pipe, P. (1997). *Analyzing performance problems, or you really oughta-wanna*. Atlanta, GA: The Center for Effective Performance, Inc.

O'Brien, R. M., Dickinson, A. M., & Rosow, R. P. (Eds.). (1982). *Industrial behavior modification*. New York: Pergamon Press.

Rummler, G. A., & Brache, A. P. (2012). *Improving performance: How to manage the white space in the organizational chart* (3rd ed.). San Francisco: Josey-Bass.

REFERENCES

Bailey, J. S. (1998). *A dozen diagnostic questions*. Unpublished manuscript.

Bailey, J. S., & Austin, J. (1996). Productivity in the workplace. In M. A. Mattaini & B. A. Thyer (Eds.), *Finding solutions to social problems: Behavioral strategies for change* (pp. 179–200). Hoboken, NJ: John Wiley & Sons, Ltd. https://doi.org/10.1037/10217-007

Bailey, J. S., & Burch, M. R. (2018). *Research methods in applied behavior analysis* (2nd ed.). New York: Routledge, Inc.

Conrad, D. A. (2016, April). The theory of value-based payment incentives and their application to health care. *Health Services Research, 50*(s2), 2057–2089. https://doi.org/10.1111/1475-6773.12408

Daniels, A. C. (2000). *Bringing out the best in people.* New York: McGraw-Hill.

Daniels, A. C., & Bailey, J. (2014). *Performance management: Changing behavior that drives organizational effectiveness* (5th ed.). Atlanta: Performance Management Publications.

Ditzian, K., Wilder, D. A., King, A., & Tanz, J. (2015). An evaluation of the performance diagnostic checklist—Human Services to assess an employee performance problem in a center-based autism treatment facility. *Journal of Applied Behavior Analysis, 48*, 199–203.

Gilbert, T. F. (1978). *Human competence-engineering worthy performance.* New York: McGraw Hill.

Kent, R. S. (1985). *25 steps to getting performance problems off your desk . . . and out of your life*! New York: Dodd, Mead, and Company.

Mager, R. F., & Pipe, P. (1970). *Analyzing performance problems.* Belmont, CA: Fearon Publishers.

Reid, D. H. (1998). *Organizational behavior management and developmental disabilities: Accomplishments and future directions.* New York: Haworth Press.

Reid, D. H., Parsons, M. B., & Green, C. W. (2012). *The supervisor's guidebook: Evidence-based strategies for promoting work quality and enjoyment among human service staff.* Chapel Hill, NC: Professional Press.

Rodriguez, M. (2021). *Organizational behavior management: A practitioner's guide to making a positive difference.* Miami: Bueno Ventures Management Services, Inc.

15

School-Based Behavior Analysis

Dr. Jennifer L. Austin

FRESH OUT OF GRAD SCHOOL, FIRST JOB

The first thing you need to know about being a behavior analyst in schools is that there are very few problems that happen there for which behavior analysis does not offer a solution. In fact, behavior analysts have been interested in improving school practices for decades. Even B. F. Skinner (1968, 1984) was intensely interested in applying our science to make classrooms more efficient and effective learning environments. Many other behavior analysts have devoted their entire careers to advancing behavior analysis as a positive, proactive, and evidence-based solution to many of the challenges educators face today, including helping at-risk children "catch up" academically, building students' fluency in core academic competencies such as reading and math, developing classroom management strategies that can be easily integrated into school routines, and

> Behavior analysts working in schools need to be familiar with a range of strategies that will provide the roadmap to solving most of the problems they will encounter.

DOI: 10.4324/9781003265573-18

transforming school cultures to create more positive environments for students and their teachers.

The Good Behavior Game (GBG; Joslyn, Austin, Donaldson, & Vollmer, 2020), Direct Instruction (DI; Stockard, 2021), fluency-building (Gist & Bulla, 2020), Active Student Responding (ASR; Twyman & Heward, 2018), and school-wide Positive Behavior Interventions and Supports (PBIS; Horner & Sugai, 2015) are just a few of the school-specific strategies from the behavioral literature. Given the volume of behavior analytic research in education, behavior analysts working in schools need to be familiar with a range of strategies that will provide the roadmap to solving most of the problems they will encounter. Perhaps you were fortunate enough to have learned about some of these strategies in your graduate program, which will give you a leg up as you begin to work in classrooms. Even so, as with any application of behavior analysis, you will likely need to do some independent reading to ensure you are up-to-speed on the literature for specific strategies. As a new behavior analyst, you are not expected to be an expert at everything. However, as you progress as a professional, you should be updating and expanding your behavior analytic toolkit. Even if you are a BCBA, it is a good idea to identify a colleague who is an expert in working in schools to provide guidance and supervision for your work as a new professional.

Recognizing the Right Target

Your graduate program and practicum experiences likely instilled in you the importance of analyzing behavior at the individual level, which means identifying socially important target behaviors, conducting a functional assessment or analysis of those behaviors, and then implementing and monitoring a highly individualized intervention plan to reduce behaviors that interfere with success and increase behaviors that promote it. This is a good and ethical practice and will hold you in good stead when you are asked to support a student whose behavior is limiting his or her success at school. However, imagine that you have a referral for Thomas, who is in first grade and has been described by his teacher as "one of the most challenging students I've ever tried to teach." You have planned to do an informant assessment with his teacher, Mrs. Hayes, who has suggested a meeting when the children are at recess. You show up a bit early, give Mrs. Hayes a quick wave and smile as you enter the classroom, and then find a small chair in the back of the room where you can do a bit of observation prior to your meeting. You hope your brief observation will provide some context for your upcoming discussion about Thomas, as you are hoping to see some of the behaviors firsthand. The problem is that you can't identify which student Thomas is because nearly every student in the classroom is engaging in some type of disruptive behavior. You observe children chasing each other around the classroom, playing with materials that have nothing to do with the lesson, throwing pencils at one another, making silly noises, and falling dramatically out of their chairs. In a class of at least 25 students, only a handful seem to be engaged with the lesson (and you are not quite sure how, as the classroom is so noisy that you feel like you need an aspirin). When the children are outside and you finally have a chance to say a proper hello to Mrs. Hayes, her first comment to you is, "If I didn't have a mortgage to pay, I'd quit my job."

Hopefully, at this point, you would realize that your conversation is no longer going to be exclusively about Thomas. You have a teacher in crisis, who is burned out and feeling defeated. You also have an entire classroom of students (even the ones who are doing the right thing) who will benefit from a more peaceful and organized classroom. Proceeding with plans to complete a functional behavior assessment and individualized intervention for Thomas is unlikely to be effective for several reasons, chief among them being that the teacher, who is clearly overwhelmed, likely will not be able to implement it with integrity. Further, attempting to facilitate successful intervention in a classroom as chaotic as this one is going to make your (and the teacher's) job more difficult. It is possible that Thomas *will* need an individualized behavior plan, but before you proceed down that road, you need to prepare the classroom for successful implementation and determine whether a classroom-wide intervention might solve Thomas's problems. Therefore, as a new behavior analyst, you should be equipped to offer guidance and coaching on classroom management.

Being familiar with the Good Behavior Game (GBG) will be a massive help in situations like the one encountered with Mrs. Hayes. Based on an interdependent group contingency, the GBG helps teachers to remember to use core classroom management strategies, including setting clear expectations for behavior, providing consistent feedback on the degree to which students are meeting those expectations, and ensuring that good behavior leads to positive consequences. Students are divided into teams and then work as a team to meet classroom expectations (i.e., follow the rules of the game). The original version of the GBG is arranged so that points are awarded to teams if anyone on the team breaks a rule, so the goal is to earn less than a certain number of points. A revised version of the game often referred to as the Caught Being Good Game (CBGG; Wright & McCurdy, 2012) awards points to teams for following rules (i.e., it uses a DRO schedule). In the CBGG, teams win if they meet a particular point threshold. The beauty of both the GBG and the CBGG is that they are packaged as games, which makes it easy for teachers to remember to employ classroom management essentials. Games can (and should) be played multiple times per day and can be adapted to different settings (e.g., playground, cafeteria). It is also worth noting that the GBG and CBGG are effective across age ranges (from preschool to high school), and they have excellent treatment acceptability. They also are relatively robust to procedural integrity compromises, which makes them an excellent choice for busy classrooms. For a summary of recent research on the GBG, see Joslyn, Donaldson, Austin, and Vollmer (2019). For a clinician's guide to using the GBG, see Joslyn et al. (2020).

Poor instruction within a well-managed classroom won't support students to achieve their potential.

Although honing your skills as a classroom management coach is essential to your consulting repertoire, it is important to remember that good classroom management isn't always enough to ensure a productive learning environment. Poor instruction within a well-managed classroom won't support students to achieve their potential. Although there are many factors that influence the effectiveness of instruction, getting students involved in the process is an essential component. Active Student Responding (ASR, States, Detrich, & Keyworth, 2019) and fluency-building strategies are important elements of your school consultation toolkit. For example, response cards (an ASR strategy) involve prompting all students to respond to the teacher's questions simultaneously. Students can use small whiteboards to write their responses or use colored cards that correspond to different multiple-choice response options. There are even high-tech response clickers (usually referred to as Classroom Response Systems; Fies & Marshall, 2006), which display a graph of all students' responses directly to the teacher's electronic whiteboard or PowerPoint® presentation. Response cards offer the opportunity for all students to respond to each question, rather than the traditional system of hand-raising, in which only a few students typically respond. The advantage of this approach is obvious—the more opportunities there are to respond, the more opportunities there are to learn. Equally important is that it provides real-time feedback to the teacher, so she can identify struggling students and offer support before they practice mistakes when completing their independent classwork or homework.

Improving Existing Practices

As you work in schools, it is likely you will encounter a range of practices that bear some resemblance to the strategies you learned about in grad school. For example, many schools use some sort of token economy to motivate students or manage behavior. However, you might find that there are some errors in the ways these systems are used that make them less effective than they could be.

For example, you might notice that there don't appear to be clear or consistent rules about earning tokens, or response cost is overused, or there are long delays to accessing back-up reinforcers, or that tokens aren't awarded with any regularity. Your knowledge of the importance of motivating operations, contingency, and contiguity in predicting the reinforcing effects of stimuli will help you adjust these systems to maximize their impact. Sometimes it is not necessary to reinvent the wheel; offering advice on how to tweak existing strategies might preclude the need for new systems, which often require more training and resources to get off the ground.

Another strategy that you might observe in schools is time-out. Although time-out has been researched for decades, studies aimed specifically at improving the ways we use time-out has seen a resurgence in recent years. For example, Donaldson, Vollmer, Yakich, and Van Camp (2013) found that you can reduce noncompliance to going to time-out by shortening time-out duration when children agree to go immediately. They also found that requiring the absence of problem behavior as a condition of release from time-out was no more effective than allowing children to leave when their time was up (i.e., even if they had not behaved well during the time-out; Donaldson & Vollmer, 2011). Taken together, this research shows how we can implement time-out in ways that effectively reduce problem behaviors, but also limit the time children spend in time-out—which frees up more time for meaningful activities in the classroom. For a review of the recent research on time-out, see Corralejo, Jensen, Greathouse, and Ward (2018).

> Appeals to relying on evidence as a rationale for using behavior analytic strategies are often ignored.

Navigating Obstacles

Working in schools as a behavior analyst can be incredibly reinforcing. Seeing children become more successful learners and helping stressed-out teachers reclaim their confidence and love of teaching is powerful. However, you also need to be prepared for the myriad of obstacles schools might place on your path to success. Probably one of the biggest frustrations you will encounter is that schools do not always operate according to solid evidence regarding the best ways of teaching or promoting positive behavior. School decision-makers might be more persuaded by dogma or the latest educational fads than they are by credible, peer-reviewed research. They also might have different ideas about what constitutes good research; for example, they might equate the evidence provided by a case study with that produced by a randomized controlled trial. In this environment, appeals to relying on evidence as a rationale for using behavior analytic strategies are often ignored.

A related obstacle is that it might be difficult for teachers to see the value in repeated measures of behavior, which are a mainstay of behavior analytic research and practice. Teachers are used to assessing performance, but their measures typically employ permanent products rather than the real-time recording of behavior. And let's face it—teachers simply do not have the time to record data in the way a behavior analyst would, so don't be disappointed when the partial interval recording data sheet you left with the teacher is never completed.

Most teachers know that evidence-based practices are important, but they might not have learned how to identify good evidence in their teacher education programs. You can help them acquire this repertoire by sharing some articles about the strategies you suggest, but choose wisely. Teachers are busy people, so don't overload them with a list of references or send a copy of an article that you yourself had to read a dozen times before you understood it. Keep it simple. Perhaps choose one article and highlight the most important parts that informed what you decided to do in their classroom or for a particular student. If you want teachers to collect data to help assess treatment effectiveness, keep that simple, too. Sometimes a very blunt instrument (e.g., momentary time sampling at the end of each lesson) is better than a more refined data collection system that never gets used. Of course, teacher data collection should not supplant your ongoing monitoring, but it can be a very helpful part of evaluating how well interventions are working from the teacher's perspective. Also, be sure to share your data with the teacher to model data-based decision-making.

Another obstacle that you will quickly need to learn to deal with is the loss of control over intervention implementation. Your role in the school will likely be that of a consultant or coach, so you will be handing over strategy implementation to the teacher or a paraprofessional. Unfortunately, it is not uncommon to come back a few days later to find an unrecognizable version of the strategy you recommended, complete with feedback from a frustrated teacher that it isn't working.

> A great intervention that never gets implemented is not a great intervention.

As behavior analysts, we know that behavior takes time to change. However, for a teacher who is desperate for improved behavior and more successful students, expectations for how quickly a strategy should work might not be realistic. If the teacher implements your strategy and does not see immediate results, that effectively puts her intervening behavior on extinction. Extinction produces response variability, which is why your original strategy now has extra components (or might have lost essential ones). Granted, sometimes teachers make excellent suggestions about how to adapt a strategy, which can increase effectiveness and improve contextual fit. However, the time to discuss those adaptations is in the planning process, not after the teacher has independently decided to use them. Incorporating the teacher's suggestions (and her non-negotiables) when you are planning the intervention can help facilitate buy-in and treatment acceptability. Sometimes this process results in an intervention that is not exactly what you would have prescribed if you were the only one calling the shots. However, it is important to focus on what is feasible and acceptable to the teacher, as he or she is the one who will have to implement the strategy. A great intervention that never gets implemented is not a great intervention.

Facilitating intervention success also involves being a good coach. Make sure the game plan is written out in non-technical language and that it includes a task analysis for implementation. Also consider writing a troubleshooting guide (i.e., if this particular thing goes wrong, do this) so the teacher can carry on when faced with common pitfalls. Take time to review the plan face-to-face, rather than emailing it and asking the teacher to contact you with any questions. Consider using behavioral skills training (BST), and if possible, be in the classroom on the first day of implementation to help coach the teacher through the first few plays.

One additional obstacle worth mentioning is the general resistance to behavior analysis in education. Despite the wealth of contributions behavior analysts have made to school improvement, it is not uncommon to encounter school personnel who believe behavior analysis has no place in modern education. Rather than getting on the defensive, take a deep breath and listen. Often you will find that these perceptions come from fundamental misunderstandings of the science and its ethical application. They might also arise from a bad experience with a behavior analyst who disregarded the views of others and wasn't a good coach or team player. Be careful not to make the same mistakes. Remember that you are an ambassador for behavior analysis, and what people think of behavior analysis might come down to what they think of you.

YOUNG PROFESSIONAL (3–5 YEARS)

Now that you have some experience under your belt, you will have lots of data (and stories to tell) about addressing challenging behaviors at both the individual and classroom level. You also will have learned some lessons about what not to do, which will have broadened your problem-solving skills. All in all, you will have built a repertoire that will help you tackle a more diverse range of problems. Although you likely will continue to consult with individual teachers, you also will be prepared to deliver larger scale trainings to groups of teachers or entire schools. Waiting until you've accrued more "front line" experience before attempting to train large groups is a good strategy, as it makes you better prepared with data-based answers to the range of questions and problems your audience might raise.

MID-CAREER (6–10 YEARS)

You might find that much of your role in the early years of school consulting is that of a firefighter. In other words, you spend most of your time reacting to problems rather than actively preventing them from occurring. As you add more and more skills to your behavior analytic repertoire, you will be ready to facilitate more system-wide changes in schools. That is, you will have the skills and experience to shift a reactive culture to one focused on prevention and more efficient use of resources. School-wide Positive Behavior Interventions and Supports (PBIS; Horner & Sugai, 2015) provides a framework for enacting these types of changes.

Based on public health models, the PBIS framework was developed on the assumption that all students will benefit from preventative strategies implemented across the school. These include such things as setting clear expectations for behavior, delivering high-quality systems to positively reinforce those behaviors, using evidence-based teaching strategies, and ensuring good home-school communication systems. Collectively, these preventative strategies are referred to as tier one interventions. Those students who continue to struggle at tier-one advance to tier-two, which provides more focused, evidence-based interventions for specific types of problems. For instance, students might receive social skills instruction, academic tutoring, or use a Check-In/Check-Out system to provide more targeted expectations, feedback, and reinforcement. Students whose behavior or academic needs cannot be met by tier-two advance to tier-three, which involves an FBA and highly individualized intervention planning. However, by taking the preventative approach facilitated by the lower tiers, typically less than 5% of the entire student body will require tier three intervention. Because of your years of experience facilitating both classroom and individual intervention strategies, you will be well placed to support schools in building multi-tiered intervention systems.

SENIOR BEHAVIOR ANALYST

Later in your career, you might find that you do less and less work directly in classrooms. Instead, you probably will be coordinating large teams of BCBAs and RBTs to deliver consultation and intervention support across multiple schools or school districts. Because you will likely have a reputation as someone who is effective, professional, and supportive, school leaders will seek you out to help them transform the ways they deal with problem behavior and promote student success. However, be careful not to become too far removed from the everyday experiences of teachers and students. Taking a few cases, yourself (rather than delegating them to your team) will help you stay close to the issues that are important to teachers and the children they teach.

SUMMARY

This chapter described some of the ways that behavior analysts might work in schools to improve outcomes for students and their teachers. Behavior problems are rife in classrooms, despite a raft of policies to tackle them. Teachers often find themselves overwhelmed by the sheer number of behavioral issues they deal with on a day-to-day basis, which can lead to stress and burnout. And it is not just teachers who suffer; students with behavior problems are at risk for poorer academic outcomes, and persistent disruptions can adversely affect the learning environment for everyone in the class. Although the behavior analytic literature has provided a wealth of effective strategies, schools can be challenging environments for both new and experienced behavior analysts. Decision-making often is not data-based and prevailing beliefs about how children should learn can create barriers to the adoption of behavior analytic strategies and the degree to which they are implemented with integrity. However, it is our job to advocate for evidence-based practices as solutions to both academic and behavioral challenges.

REFERENCES

Corralejo, S. M., Jensen, S. A., Greathouse, A. D., & Ward, L. E. (2018). Parameters of time-out: Research update and comparison to parenting programs, books, and online recommendations. *Behavior Therapy*, *49*(1), 99–12. https://doi.org/10.1016/j.beth.2017.09.005

Donaldson, J. M., & Vollmer, T. R. (2011). An evaluation and comparison of time-out procedures with and without release contingencies. *Journal of Applied Behavior Analysis*, *44*, 693–705. https://doi.org/10.1901/jaba.2011.44-693

Donaldson, J. M., Vollmer, T. R., Yakich, T. M., & Van Camp, C. (2013). Effects of a reduced time-out interval on compliance with the time-out instruction. *Journal of Applied Behavior Analysis*, *46*, 369–378. https://doi.org/10.1002/jaba.40

Fies, C., & Marshall, J. (2006). Classroom response systems: A review of the literature. *Journal of Science Education and Technology*, *15*, 101–109. https://doi.org/10.1007/s10956-006-0360-1

Gist, C., & Bulla, A. J. (2020). A systematic review of frequency building and precision teaching with school-aged children. *Journal of Behavioral Education*, 1–26. https://doi.org/10.1007/s10864-020-09404-3

Horner, R. H., & Sugai, G. (2015). School-wide PBIS: An example of applied behavior analysis implemented at a scale of social importance. *Behavior Analysis in Practice*, *8*, 80–85. https://doi.org/10.1007/s40617-015-0045-4

Joslyn, P. R., Austin, J. L., Donaldson, J. M., & Vollmer, T. R. (2020). A practitioner's guide to the good behavior game. *Behavior Analysis: Research and Practice*, *20*, 219–235. https://doi.org/10.1037/bar0000199

Joslyn, P. R., Donaldson, J. M., Austin, J. L., & Vollmer, T. R. (2019). The good behavior game: A brief review. *Journal of Applied Behavior Analysis*, *52*, 811–815. http://hvar.is/upload/4/SFX/sfx.gif

Skinner, B. F. (1968). *The technology of teaching*. Washington, DC: New Appleton-Century-Crofts.

Skinner, B. F. (1984). The shame of American education. *American Psychologist*, *39*(9), 947–954. https://doi.org/10.1037/0003-066X.39.9.947

States, J., Detrich, R., & Keyworth, R. (2019). *Active student responding (ASR) overview*. Oakland, CA: The Wing Institute. Retrieved from www.winginstitute.org/instructional-delivery-student-respond

Stockard, J. (2021). Building a more effective, equitable, and compassionate educational system: The role of direct instruction. *Perspectives on Behavior Science*, *44*(2), 147–167. https://doi.org/10.1007/s40614-021-00287-x

Twyman, J. S., & Heward, W. L. (2018). How to improve student learning in every classroom now. *International Journal of Educational Research*, *87*, 78–90. https://doi.org/10.1016/j.ijer.2016.05.007

Wright, R. A., & McCurdy, B. L. (2012). Class-wide positive behavior support and group contingencies: Examining a positive variation of the good behavior game. *Journal of Positive Behavior Interventions*, *14*, 173–180. https://doi.org/10.1177/1098300711421008

Unit

Four

Vital Work Habits

After graduating with a master's degree and working for seven years, a BCBA went to visit her college professor.

> I really loved our graduate program. The faculty and other students were wonderful. When I started my first job, I felt so well-trained in ABA. I just can't thank you enough. But if I had to give some feedback, I'd say what I didn't learn in school was the soft skills that go along with being a professional behavior analyst. I needed a lot of help with time management, and I was shaky as a public speaker—maybe because our professors did all the talking.
>
> I also needed guidance on becoming a trusted professional, and how to network with other behavior analysts and become a strong part of a team. For the first few years of my job, I had so much on my plate it would have been helpful if I had some tips

DOI: 10.4324/9781003265573-19

on dealing with stress, maybe in the professional issues class. I'm doing better now.

Thank you again for all that you taught me, I love being a behavior analyst.

16

Time Management the Behavioral Way

Take five minutes to plan your day.

—Brian A. Iwata

FRESH OUT OF GRAD SCHOOL, FIRST JOB

Behavior analysts are busy people who are generally in great demand by clients, stakeholders, teachers, parents, administrators, corporate executives, and others looking to improve the lives of their clientele. A typical day for a behavior analyst might start early with a meeting with a principal to iron out issues with a student who is not showing improvement despite a thorough IEP. The BCBA then rushes to consult with a teacher who is not on board with a new behavior plan. In the meantime, her cell phone has pinged three times, indicating she has text messages to return as soon as she gets a break which will probably be in her car on the way to a client's house to supervise a brand new RBT. And so it goes throughout the week, with the behavior analyst rushing to avoid being late because traffic was heavy, or a client was having a meltdown. The requirements of the job also mean keeping track of billable hours, sometimes in quarter-hour intervals, completing progress reports, conducting numerous supervision sessions, and making presentations to school teams developing individualized education programs.

DOI: 10.4324/9781003265573-20

Learning to plan your day and manage your time is an essential skill for the successful behavior analyst, and there are many, many distractions that will be competing for your attention. As you reflect on your progress at the end of the day, you realize your 30-minute meeting with the principal went well because you were able to give her the advice she needed on how to handle an unresponsive child. In one of the IMs from your BCaBA, you were able to suggest a *JABA* article to support a new behavior-change intervention, and you regrettably had to turn down an invite from a friend who wanted you to meet after work. As much fun as it would have been to catch up, this was bad timing because you have an important report due the next day pertaining to a client custody situation for which you could end up testifying in court.

Core Time Management Skills

Basic time management should include the following five key elements Spica.com. (n.d.):

1. Planning

For behavior analysts, this will usually start with a weekly calendar (see Figure 16.1) where you outline your standing appointments, routine meetings, supervision visits, writing deadlines, and planned conferences. Following this you will need to drill down for each day to fill in the details as to whom you are meeting with and where, the purpose of the meeting, and the anticipated start and stop time including necessary travel from your base to the location. If you are working with in-home clients who occasionally cancel an appointment you will need to plan make-up time to fill these hours.

2. Decision Making and Prioritizing

We recommend the *Getting Things Done* (GTD) model by David Allen (Allen, 2015) which is described next. Basically, you will need to take each request, email, phone call, and instant message and

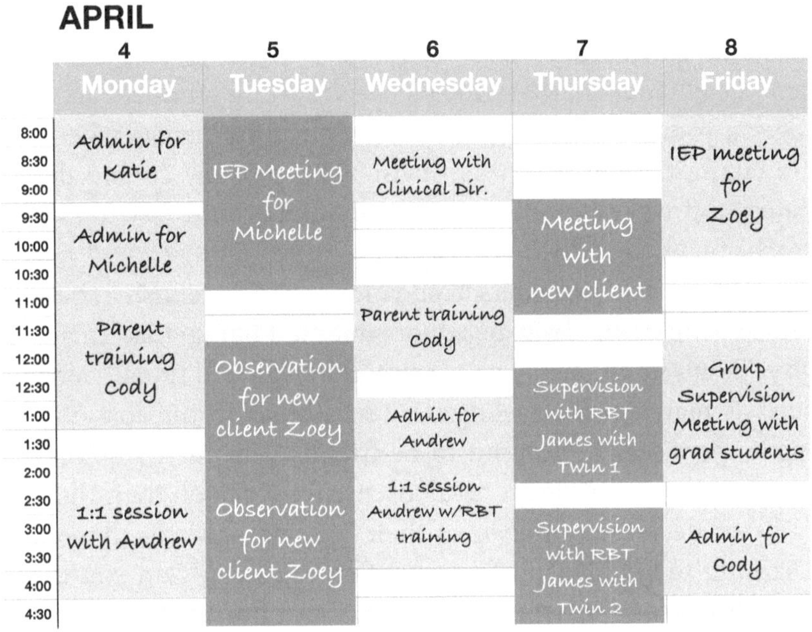

Figure 16.1 This figure shows a weekly calendar of To-Do items and meetings.

determine if you need to act on it immediately or whether you can hand it off to someone else, postpone until a later date, or determine if it does not require a response at all. Since most of the decisions will involve human behavior, your priorities in determining how and when you will respond can be critical. Making quick assessments of a situation and knowing exactly how to respond are part of the job of being a professional behavior analyst. An urgent call from a distressed RBT in a problematic home will likely take precedence over a standing meeting with the clinical director, and some emails sent to you on a weekend may have to wait until Monday.

3. Setting Boundaries and Saying "No"

Informing clients that you do not take calls during your time off is a good example of setting boundaries. In addition to calls from clients, there may be other calls that involve not only clients but colleagues, direct reports, and administrators. While you should set boundaries, you should always have an "In case of an emergency, call (consultant's name) at the following number . . ." message on your voice mail or as an autoreply to your email when you are taking time off. Your supervisor and possibly certain designated staff will have your cell phone number or a way to always reach you.

Clients and stakeholders would often like to establish a friendly relationship with their behavior analyst hoping that this will give them more personal service, provide additional benefits such as marriage counseling or even a break in the cost of billing. Supervisees often want to be friends with their supervisors to possibly prevent direct no-nonsense feedback on their therapy skills or decrease criticism of their missing sessions altogether. Learning to say "No" to friendly offers such as, "Can you come to my wedding?" personal requests, "Can I borrow your car?" or questionable business offers, "Would you like to get in on the real estate deal of a lifetime?" represent a test of your interpersonal skills, as well as your ability to fluently use autoclitics (Skinner, 1957, Ch. 12). As Skinner describes in great detail, how you use certain phrases, can make all the difference in the response from your listener, e.g., "I appreciate that you think I might be able to give you some advice about your partner's behavior, but I am not qualified to do so. This is beyond my scope of practice," or "I am so sorry, but I am on a doctor-prescribed low-carb diet, and I don't eat sugar. But I would like to donate to the Girl Scouts."

4. Delegating Tasks

Learning how to delegate certain tasks to your direct reports can make all the difference in how much time you have to complete your major assignments. RBTs can be trained to graph their own data and BCaBAs can be coached to cover the routine supervision of trainees. This will leave you time to work on serious client-related behavior problems requiring a high-level understanding of current research and billing codes. You must, however, not delegate tasks that supervisees are prohibited from doing such as writing behavior plans, training parents, and administering assessments.

5. Build Your Own Time Management System

After you review the GTD system or other similar systems, you will need to adopt those features that fit your type of work and your desired lifestyle. The GTD system, for example, was designed around the premise of a person working at a desk in a busy office. This contrasts with the job of behavior analysts who are largely mobile and probably do most of their required paperwork (now digital) on a laptop wherever they can find a quiet spot during the day. Most of your day will be spent interacting with clients, stakeholders, and supervisees and your decision-making, prioritizing, setting boundaries and delegating will probably be done in the moment on the run. You may have to record your decisions and alterations to daily plans on a voice recorder to be sorted out later in the day.

Time Management the Behavioral Way Allen's system covers all the important aspects of time and project management, and we highly recommend his book to all new behavioral consultants. There is one feature that is not included that may be important to behavior analysts who are interested in the motivational aspects of work completion. Allen assumed that task completion itself is a natural reinforcer. It may be for many people, but for some, there is a need for something else, such as a *consequence*, to keep moving ahead with tasks that are boring, arduous, or unfulfilling. To fill the gap, we suggest a basic behavioral procedure with which you are no doubt already acquainted and that is the *Premack Principle*. The Premack Principle (see Figure 16.2) basically states that more-probable behaviors will reinforce less-probable behaviors. During the week, your behavior analysis work will involve supervising trainees, RBTs and BCaBAs. You may also be doing direct therapy that is likely to be quite structured with a few clients (see Figures 16.3 and 16.4). Your weekends may not be completely filled with leisure as you will have regular chores and some case assignments to complete. Using the Premack Principle can help you complete these "not fun" tasks that you might otherwise just put off until another day. Developing a habit of pairing the completion of a task such as paying the bills or cleaning out the garage with a reinforcing event like working in the garden or going out for pizza with your friends will give you a great deal of satisfaction.

> By using a time management system, you will find that you accomplish more, have less stress, and can fully enjoy your leisure time since you don't have uncompleted tasks hanging over your weekends and holidays.

We also recommend the simple act of putting a distinctive checkmark by each item completed on your To-Do list so that at the end of the day you can visually scan your calendar and see how much you have accomplished.

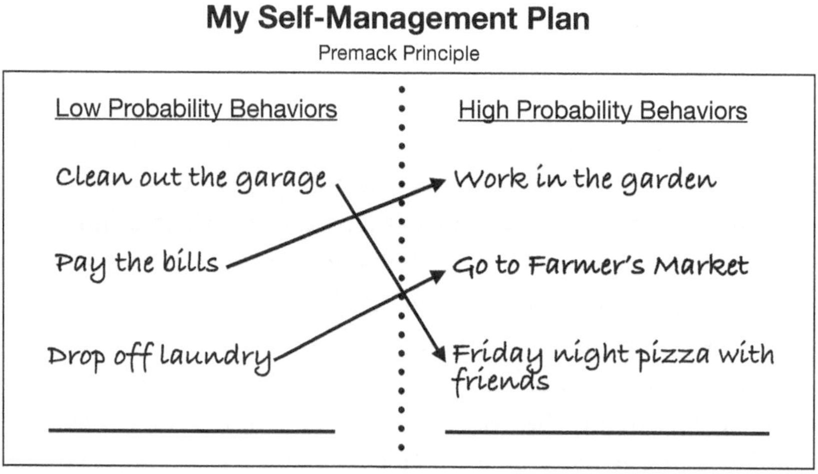

Figure 16.2 This figure shows an example of using the Premack Principle to reinforce daily work activities.

Wednesday April 13, 2022

TO DO TODAY	APPOINTMENTS & MEETINGS	WORK RECORD	TIME	EXPENSES
☑ Finish update for Clay	IEP Meeting for Michele	Meeting 8:00-10:00	8:00 9:00 2hr/ 10:00 30 min 11:00	
☑ Enter/ review data Michele	Meeting with Cody caregivers/ stakeholders to discuss progress	Meeting 10:30-1:30 Admin 2:00-2:30	12:00 1:00 2:00 30 3:00 min 4:00 1hr	Supplies for new client
☐ Finish feedback form for RBTs	Meeting with new RBT Janet	Supervision in home 3:00-4:00	5:00 6:00 7:00 8:00	

Figure 16.3 This figure shows an example of a BCBA's To-Do list and planning notes for one day of service delivery.

YOUNG PROFESSIONAL (3–5 YEARS)

If you have been able to settle on a time management system that works for you, you should begin to see how important it is for your success as a professional. By using a time management system, you will find that you accomplish more, have less stress, and can fully enjoy your leisure time since you don't have uncompleted tasks hanging over your weekends and holidays. Now is the time to be an explicit role model for your RBTs and trainees with your time management prowess and to develop methods of teaching them the power of managing their time wisely. As a supervisor, you can require your supervisees and trainees to develop To-Do lists (Gawande, 2009) for their daily assignments and coach them on the value of using the Premack Principle during their time off. During supervision, you can have supervisees take notes on your feedback. Put your comments and suggestions in bullet point format for guidance prior to the next supervision session. If supervisees can demonstrate mastery of each item, you can prompt them to check off the items and compliment their success.

MID-CAREER (6–10 YEARS)

At mid-career, time management will have become a background activity that is so automatic you almost do not notice it. If you are off on the weekends, on Sunday evenings you will find yourself reviewing your monthly and weekly calendars to see what you have committed to and where you need to be each day. Since you will likely be operating at the mid-management level or higher in your organization, the types of meetings you will take, or run, will have a more significant impact on a larger number of people. The challenges on your time will no doubt be greater and your finesse in deflecting these without offending people will have greatly improved. Most likely the biggest change you will see at this level is your constant need to plan your schedule in fine detail and delegate tasks to others under your supervision.

SENIOR BEHAVIOR ANALYST

When you reach this level in any organization, time management becomes largely a matter of prioritizing and focused decision-making. Your time will be so valuable that your company will probably provide you with an assistant who can manage your calendar and act as a gatekeeper so that you are only dealing with the most important decisions that need to be made in the company. As a CEO or chairman of the board, your assistant will prompt you about upcoming meetings and deadlines that must be met for reports to be reviewed or talks to be presented at conferences.

SUMMARY

This chapter on time management presented a variety of ways that busy behavior analysts can organize their work to maximize their productivity. Five key areas were explained in some detail. These include planning the overall schedule, drilling down to organize the weekly or monthly schedules, approaching the work in a way that is streamlined and efficient, setting boundaries, and learning to say “No” to requests that will prevent you from completing your main objectives. Two additional suggestions included delegating tasks to others who can support your work and building a personalized time management system to suit your personal style and professional objectives. Insights into how professionals with years of experience are likely to manage their time were also presented.

REFERENCES

Allen, D. (2015). *Getting things done: The art of stress-free productivity*. New York: Penguin.

Gawande, A. (2009). *The checklist manifesto: How to get things right*. New York: Henry Holt & Co.

Skinner, B. F. (1957). *Verbal behavior*. Englewood Cliffs, NJ: Prentice Hall.

Spica.com. (n.d.). *Core time management skills and how to develop them*. Retrieved April 3, 2022, from www.spica.com/blog/time-management-skills

17

Become a Trusted Professional

Trust takes years to build, seconds to break, and forever to repair.

—Anonymous

FRESH OUT OF GRAD SCHOOL, FIRST JOB

An enthusiastic first-year graduate student in an applied behavior analysis program was looking forward to starting her internship and learning new skills. She was anxious to meet her clinical supervisor, who had excellent behavioral skills and who had promised to teach her everything she needed to know to be a successful behavior analyst. Full of excitement, the student went to her first scheduled meeting with the clinical supervisor. The supervisor started the meeting by telling the student she needed to adjust her schedule of school visits to match the supervisor's schedule. The student was then informed she would receive training, observations by the supervisor, and feedback once a week, starting on the following Monday. This was great news. After all, the supervisor had 15 years of experience and came with a reputation as a behavioral clinician who could solve nearly any problem. When Monday came, the supervisor rushed into the room more than 30 minutes late. He blurted out, "I really don't have time to work with you today. Just show me what you know how to do." The supervisor was reading and

DOI: 10.4324/9781003265573-21

returning emails on his cell phone during the entire "supervision." At the end of the session, he said, "You're doing fine," and that was it. The following week, the supervisor called the student five minutes prior to their appointment and said he was canceling, muttering that his wife was out of town, and he had to "take Jenny to the doctor, she's running a fever." The following week the supervisor did not show up at all and did not even bother to call. The student sent a text to the supervisor and left email messages that were not returned. Two more weeks went by with no contact from the supervisor. The semester was now half over, and the student had received no training and no feedback. In the eighth week, the supervisor showed up on time, said, "How's it going?" and proceeded to make two calls on his cell phone. He didn't apologize for being absent or offer any explanation. When he left the building, he said, "Okay, see you next week" and hurried off.

Unfortunately, this is a true story involving a supervisor who appeared to do everything he could to actively build a *lack* of trust. He may have had very good reasons for missing sessions or being late, but the student would rightfully be justified in having very little trust in this supervisor going forward.

Achieving Trust

Trust is hard to achieve and comes only through hard work over time. To earn the trust of others, you need to demonstrate a steady, consistent temperament and be honest and reliable (Harvard Business School Press, 2005). "Trust me" is perhaps the single most overused expression in our culture and, of course, is often a dead giveaway that the speaker is certainly *not* to be trusted with anything. True trust is earned over time as you engage in your daily activities with colleagues and clients. You promise to meet a person at a certain time, and, despite the horrific weather, you show up. You listen to the plight of a friend who shares a confidence, and you *never* reveal it to anyone even if asked. You express your strong support of evidence-based treatments, and despite pressure and pleadings from a client, you refuse to endorse a fad treatment. All of these are examples of ways in which trust is gained over time.

It seems that in every office, there is a jokester who will say anything to get a rise out of people. The jokester's inappropriate comments, which can be crude or insensitive, are usually followed by "Just kidding." Individuals who engage in such antics may be amusing, and they might help lighten up the day in the workplace, but they are unlikely to be trusted by those around them. People who can't get the fooling around under control are often considered gossips, cranks, pranksters, and lightweights, and their occasional expressions of commitment and sincerity are not taken seriously. A related concern for the behavior analyst who wants to become a trusted professional is the adage, "You are known by the company you keep," which is clearly relevant here.

> You do not need to offer an opinion on every topic or push your ideas at every meeting . . . being somewhat reserved and perhaps reluctant to be drawn into the fray is one sign of a person who wants to be taken seriously.

Getting Started Building Trust

The first step to *becoming* a trusted professional is to be able to identify the characteristics of these rare individuals. A trusted professional is a person who, above all else, is honest in their dealings with others, is fair in their assessment of difficult situations (i.e., unbiased, not judgmental), and does not place blame but rather uses their behavior analytic skills to find workable solutions that are fair to all parties. In behavioral terms, we say a trusted professional is a person who responds to the available evidence and is consistent in that regard. Subjectively, the trusted individual is steady, calm, reserved, deliberate, thoughtful, consistent, reliable, confidential, dependable, loyal, and steadfast. If you look around and ask, "Who are my colleagues who have these characteristics?" you will be headed in the right direction. Once you identify a person who is trustworthy, you will want to seek that person out, begin to observe the person in various situations, and, if possible, associate yourself with this professional. It is likely that these trusted professionals are in a leadership position, have considerable visibility, and are no doubt busy. You don't want to become a pest or insult them with flattery; quietly observing how they handle difficult situations is your first best strategy. If you can be part of a working group with this person and learn first-hand how this individual looks at the world and sizes up issues as they arise, you will learn a great deal.

TRUST

In his great little book *Building Trust* (Bracey, 2002), Bracey outlined five steps spelling out TRUST. He delineated the following steps a professional can take to build trust:

Be **T**ransparent
Be **R**esponsive
Use Caring
Be **S**incere, and
Be **T**rustworthy

BE TRANSPARENT

Bracey argued that for others to trust you, they must be able to see how you think through issues. You also should be "easily readable" to those around you. If you come up with a recommendation totally out of the blue, not connected with previous ideas or suggestions, it may be difficult for others to trust your logic or your judgment. Being able to logically think aloud about a problem so that listeners can tell that each step is logical and

> Being able to logically think aloud about a problem so that listeners can tell that each step is logical and sensible is a great way to build others' trust in your judgments.

sensible is a great way to build others' trust in your judgments. You won't have to do this with all your ideas, but it certainly helps in the beginning when you are trying to establish yourself as trustworthy.

A second method of establishing trust involves presenting "easily readable behavior" when you are dealing with people (Bracey, 2002, p. 20). Bracey said that allowing people to see how you feel about situations builds trust in the sense that they know where you stand and will not be surprised by your decisions later. Tactfully letting people know that you are pleased or unhappy with how a project is going gives them the information that they need to make corrections. They will respect you and trust you, especially if your decisions match your readable behaviors. The poker-faced administrator makes everyone uneasy because people never know where they stand with this person. Trust comes from projecting strategic openness during critical meetings.

BE RESPONSIVE

Bracey asserted that trust also comes from being responsive to those around you, that is, giving feedback in a constructive, spontaneous, and caring manner (Bracey, 2002, p. 23). We usually think of feedback as a way of changing someone's behavior, but Bracey put a different twist on this, suggesting if the purpose is to help the other person, the result will be that the individual will come to trust you. Giving positive feedback changes behavior and builds trust. Thinking more broadly about the reason we give feedback allows us to see that Bracey's observation is quite true. By shaping on someone's behavior, we are essentially saying, "I am prepared to make an investment in your future. I know that you have potential, I see that you are trying, and I am prepared to make you successful. You are worthy of feedback, and I am sure that you can improve and make a difference in the life of these clients." As behavior analysts, we often miss this interpretation of the importance of giving positive feedback to those around us. In doing so, we may have also missed the opportunity to build trust.

USE CARING

Gaining the trust of colleagues means paying attention to the subtleties of social interactions. The way in which you react to their questions, comments, or presentations can make a big difference in whether your colleagues will trust you with certain kinds of information. Making eye contact when listening, paraphrasing what they say, and letting them speak without interrupting are all ways of acknowledging other people and building trust. Being careful with your language and not putting another person on the spot if his peers or supervisors are close by is an important aspect of building trust. Saying, "I'm confused. Can you go over that again?" is much better than saying, "You're confused. I have no idea what you're talking about." Dale Carnegie addressed this issue when he said, "Let the other person save face" (Carnegie, 1981, 2011). Using this strategy is especially important if the person *is* confused because pointing this out publicly could do a lot of damage to your trust factor. Taking the time to choose your words carefully and letting others know you care about their feelings will pay off when the time comes when you need someone to go the extra mile. When asked, people who trust you will come through for you because they know that you truly appreciate their efforts.

Be Sincere

Being able to match what you show in your facial expressions and body language with what you say and what you do is the formula for creating a sincere and trusting relationship with those around you. Any efforts you make to develop trust will likely fail if you come across as insincere. Using obvious insincere flattery, smiling when you are not happy, and using flat-affect positive reinforcers such as "Good job," are all detectable by friends and colleagues and will have the reverse effect of convincing others of your sincerity. Todd Risley (1937–2007) was known

Any efforts you make to develop trust will likely fail if you come across as insincere.

as a pioneer and genius in the field of behavior analysis. Among his many contributions to the field was his work on Say—Do congruence (Risley & Hart, 1968). In Risley's research on early childhood, he showed ways of teaching taught preschoolers to tell the truth by shaping on their Say—Do behaviors. As adults, we can use the same sort of contingency on ourselves to show others they can trust us to show good judgment and make good decisions. If you are trusted, your colleagues will listen to what you have to say and follow your lead.

Be Trustworthy

Being seen by others as a trusted professional has a certain downside. If you agree to do something and fail to do so, there will be consequences. Your reputation will be damaged, and you will lose a degree of trust that will have to be regained at some future time. Once trust is lost, recovery can take a while, and the process is painful. Understanding that behaviors have consequences is not new to behavior analysts, although we are more inclined to think about this in terms of other people's behavior rather than our own. Paying attention to the small commitments that are offered every day can make a big difference in whether you are trustworthy in another person's eyes. Someone saying, "Why don't you join us for dinner after work?" is a compliment of sorts. The inviter would like to spend some after-hours time with you. When you respond with, "Sure, where?" it sounds like you'll show up. If you have no intention going to dinner but just didn't know how to say "no," you just squandered a little bit of your credibility and trustworthiness. Do this enough, and you'll get the reputation of being a person who is unreliable. A socially sensitive person might even say you lied to her or embarrassed her because she told her friends you'd be there. On the flip side is the behavior analyst who is looking to build credibility and trust by forcing herself to make small commitments to do something at a specific time. It doesn't seem to matter what the commitment is if you follow through. A minor commitment is, "I'll send you a PDF of that article. I have it on my computer at home and will send it by 8:00 p.m." In the big scheme of things, it might not matter if the person gets it tonight, tomorrow, or next week. It absolutely does matter, however, in terms of building trust. It's likely that the recipient will be somewhat surprised to receive the document right on time. If you can do this sort of trust-building exercise with all the important people in your life, both personal and professional, you'll find that they will come to see you differently from everyone else they know.

Becoming a Trusted Professional Is Essential for Behavior Analysts

The behavioral paradigm is foreign to many and contrary to that of most other professionals who work in the human services arena. A child who is disruptive in his second-grade classroom (and does so to gain attention from the teacher and peers) might have a behavior program that includes extinction for tantrums.[1] This idea is certainly contrary to what the school counselor, school psychologist, and assistant principal would likely advise. The common thinking on this type of behavior is that the child *needs* attention ("He just needs to come down to my office and talk to me about his problem."), testing, or perhaps discipline ("He just needs to come down to my office for a good talking to and maybe a few hours of in-school suspension."). If the behavior analyst consulting at this school is going to receive buy in, when it comes to working with the teacher and other professionals, he will need to have some trust (behavior) in the bank. If the behavior analyst isn't seen as a trusted professional, no one will support the program he is presenting that involves ignoring minor disruptive behaviors, especially the teacher who is on the front line in this battle for control of her classroom. Furthermore, if the behavior analyst asks the teacher, who does not like this student one bit, to consistently use differential reinforcement of other behaviors (DRO) with little Darius, he is likely to get a response such as, "Give him praise for sitting quietly? After what he just called me? I don't think so!"

One strategy for gaining trust is to quickly solve some simple problems for key people who need help. Demonstrating that you are effective will help considerably with the trust issue. What others never appreciate are a lot of excuses for why you can't help them, why a program isn't working, and why you are so hard to reach when the chips are down. Building credibility and trust every single day will result in the cooperation and support you need to implement effective programs.

YOUNG PROFESSIONAL (3–5 YEARS)

Once you have settled into your position and have established yourself as someone who can be trusted you will discover that supervisees and colleagues alike will naturally be drawn to you. This is because of your solid reputation as someone who can be trusted. Your team will run smoothly and effectively because you make it clear that you trust them to engage in professional behaviors and they trust you to guide them.

MID-CAREER (6–10 YEARS)

At this stage in your career, it will become apparent that other behavior analysts who started in the company about the time that you did have fallen by the wayside. In some of these cases, the behavior analysts could be gone at least in part because they were not trustworthy. Their direct reports realized that they could not be trusted to give honest feedback, and their inconsistency in following through on promises produced trainees who were unsure of themselves and relied on excuses to get through the day. Only trusted individuals will move up in an organization since this upward mobility brings with it increased responsibility for maintaining staff, producing consistent revenue, and enhancing the reputation of the organization in the community.

SENIOR BEHAVIOR ANALYST

Once you reach senior status in any organization the obligations are huge. As a senior behavior analyst, one role you will be asked to play is that of the trusted leader, most likely the CEO or a member of the board of directors. All the employees must trust you to make wise decisions every day that are fair and honest and raise the morale of everyone in the company. In this highly visible position, you are a role model for everyone below you. In this capacity, you will be tested every day by client crises, employee missteps, and unforeseen external events. Your steady temperament, transparency, honesty, and unshakable trustworthiness will be the marks of a true leader.

SUMMARY

This chapter describes the importance of developing trust in those with whom you work. Developing trust should begin in graduate school and then blossom on your first job as a BCBA. Behavior analysts are judged by those around them and must prove that they are trustworthy and always have the best interests of their clients in mind. Achieving trust is hard work and it requires one to demonstrate a steady temperament and honest, reliable decision-making. Never say, "Trust me" as that is a dead giveaway that you have not built-up trust slowly over time. Building trust starts with making small promises and commitments ("I'll have that to you by 8:00 a.m. tomorrow"), and then absolutely following through. If you do this over and over with larger more serious commitments, then you will achieve trust.

NOTE

1 Assume that the Board Certified Behavior Analyst® has done a proper functional analysis and determined this is an attention-maintained behavior.

REFERENCES

Bracey, H. (2002). *Building trust: How to get it! How to keep it*! Taylorsville, GA: HB Artworks.

Carnegie, D. (1981). *How to win friends and influence people*. New York: Simon & Schuster.

Carnegie, D. (2011). *How to win friends and influence people in the digital age*. New York: Simon & Schuster.

Harvard Business School Press. (2005). *Power, influence, and persuasion*. Boston: Author.

Risley, T. R., & Hart, B. (1968). Developing correspondence between the non-verbal and verbal behavior of preschool children. *Journal of Applied Behavior Analysis, 1*(4), 267–281.

18

Networking

Everyone should build their network before they need it.

—Dave Delaney[1]

FRESH OUT OF GRAD SCHOOL, FIRST JOB

Networking

What Is Networking?

Networking for the freshly minted behavior analyst is more about getting a better job and improving your working conditions rather than generating business for your company, i.e., most companies have long wait lists and they have more clients than they can possibly handle. A second and equally important purpose of networking is to develop a network of peers who can serve as trusted colleagues (see Chapter 17 this book) when you have professional questions or opportunities to discuss. So, what IS networking? Basically, it boils down to meeting people in person or online, making a positive impression,

> Networking for the freshly minted behavior analyst is more about getting a better job and improving your working conditions rather than generating business for your company.

DOI: 10.4324/9781003265573-22

sharing your interests and career goals, learning about their interests and expertise, finding some common ground, and then maintaining that relationship so that at some point in the future you will be able to discuss ethical issues (with consent from the client, of course) or a business arrangement that will be beneficial to both of you.

In-person Networking This is the best approach since you can get to know the person face-to-face, and gauge their depth of knowledge, experience, and sincerity to determine if this is someone you want to pull into your circle of friends and associates. Basically, networking is a systematic method of meeting people, finding out about them, and keeping in touch as a potential future resource. There may be times when you will be able to provide assistance (in the form of consultations, support, suggestions for resources, etc.) to someone with whom you have networked, and there will be times when people can help you. The systematic part of networking involves having an organized plan to find networking opportunities and to seek out people who might be able to help you at some point in the future.

> Networking is the most successful way of finding a meaningful job and attaining career success. 80% of professionals find networking essential to their career success, almost 100% believe that face-to-face meetings build stronger long-term relationships, and 41% want to network more often.[2]

Let's start with assumptions. We're assuming that you are a recently trained behavior analyst, perhaps starting your first job in a new city. There is a good chance that you got your job through networking—a former student who graduated from the same program as you, or someone you met at a social or networking event at a behavior analysis conference, and that person passed the information along to you. You made contact, applied, interviewed, and got the job.

It is estimated that roughly 60% of jobs are landed through networking, so you can see how important this is. Here's another example of having an organized plan for networking. Suppose you are a graduate student taking a course in ethics and professional issues and are interested in acquiring the skills necessary to become a successful consultant. As you approach graduation, you'll want to get to know a lot of people who can spread the word that you are looking for a job and that you are talented, hardworking, and reliable. To be effective in creating your network, you must first have those qualities, you must impress some important people, and you need to start building your network of people who will bring up your name if they hear of a position. You'll want to attend conferences to get the word out that you are a well-trained behavior analyst looking for work, and, of course, you'll post on your Facebook and LinkedIn platforms, send text messages, send emails, and make a few phone calls to everyone in your current network.

For networking to have any power, there must be trust and integrity on both sides.

Networking is powered by the magic of *the recommendation* from someone you know who is willing to vouch for you, and, in return, you must be willing to vouch for someone else when the time comes. For networking to have any power, there must be trust and integrity on both sides. At an Association for Behavior Analysis International meeting, the first author met a former student for breakfast. In a few short years, she had become a senior consultant at a large consulting firm. As a trusted and well-respected member of the firm, she was now able to make suggestions as to whom the firm would hire for new positions. Somewhere around the second cup of coffee, one of the first author's current students walked by and was introduced, pleasantries exchanged, and the student strode off to his table. It was a brief networking opportunity, and the first author jumped on it: "He is one of my best students, very bright, very reliable, and hardworking, and he shows initiative. I'd recommend him a year from now as a great potential new hire as a consultant." This kind of input into the network can result in someone getting the job of his dreams. It is effective, however, only when the person recommended performs up to the billing he was given. If you make a mistake and recommend someone who fails to meet expectations, then your credibility goes down—way down.

While networking at state and national conferences is important, don't forget that networking can be local as well. These are colleagues in your organization or similar organizations in your geographic area. Your goal is for them to get to know you, and vice versa, so you can create a strong local network of people to support you. The kind of support your behavior analyst contacts might provide can range from helping you think through a tough clinical case that has got you stymied, to working out a delicate supervision issue with a trainee.

NETWORKING BEHAVIORS

Appearance

Because one of your goals is to make a positive impression on someone, you need to start with your appearance. All the tips in Chapter 1 on professional etiquette apply here. At any networking opportunity, you should be well-groomed and dressed appropriately for the occasion. The appropriate dress may vary for a single event. For example, at the Association for Behavior Analysis International conference, dress may be casual for hospitality suites, but more formal for a company dinner at an expensive restaurant.

Attitude

> Put on your big smile, and stride into the room, showing confidence and a casual, relaxed attitude.

If you are new to behavior analysis and you are one of those people who is not a networking natural, the excitement and anticipation of networking might remind you of when you were a 6-year-old getting ready to attend a birthday party. You don't know what you are going to get into, but you are hopeful that you are going to have a good time. When you are networking, put on your big smile, and stride into the room, showing confidence and a casual, relaxed attitude. Once in the room, stop for a minute to size up the gathering. As a warm-up, you can begin by talking to someone you know. Then move around the room and introduce yourself to some people that you don't know.

Equipment

You don't need a lot of equipment to be successful at networking, but you will need business cards to give to others. If you are old school, you can use a pen and a small notebook to record contact and other information from your new contacts. It is most likely these days that you will put the information directly into your cell phone.

Specifics of Behavioral Networking

As you approach someone, put on your big friendly smile, and introduce yourself. A part of a business introduction used to involve a firm handshake. However, when the COVID-19 pandemic started, handshakes became a thing of the past in most business and social settings. You'll have to decide what is appropriate regarding handshakes for the setting in which you are networking.

After you introduce yourself, ask a noncontroversial and open-ended question that will get the conversation started: "This is a great event; how did you hear about it?" "What business are you in?" "This is a wonderful conference. Did you hear any good talks today?" The old rule about staying away from politics and religion is a good idea and can prevent you from offending someone. Once you get the person you'd like to meet to start talking, you can be reinforcing and demonstrate your great listening skills. This should be sincere, natural, and not contrived. If you're a behavior analyst, we hope that you like people and will truly come to enjoy hearing a new friend talk about hobbies, a recent trip, or a particular area of interest in behavior analysis.

BE CURIOUS

Don't be afraid to ask questions about what people do and their hobbies, travel, children, or dogs. If they appear to be changing the subject or choosing not to elaborate on a particular topic, you need to *pick up on the subtle cues and respond appropriately with a segue to something less controversial.*

BE A CONNECTOR

As a good networker, you should try to put people together whenever you can. If you are successful, both parties will be thankful and will at some point return the favor. During your conversation, if you realize the person you are talking to should meet someone else in the room, offer to make the introduction. Say, "I have someone I'd like you to meet," and take the person over to your friend. Give a good introduction to each: "Sarah, this is Charlotte. She's the new HR director at Bright Kids." Your goal is to make a friendly impression, find a connection for yourself or someone else, get a business card, and move on. You should not dominate the time of the person you just met, because you have many more people to meet and so does everyone else. To end the conversation, be as polite as you were in the beginning, and remember that last impressions count too. To end an interaction, you could say, "I really enjoyed meeting you. Have a great time at the conference." Ideally, you'll be able to include someone else in the conversation, so you don't have to leave a person totally alone.

NETWORKING FOLLOW-UP

This aspect of networking is not discussed very often, but this is where the payoff is for the whole networking enterprise. After the networking event (e.g., social hour, informal time to chat after a meeting), such as later that evening or early the next morning, review the business cards you accumulated and the notes you took. As you flip through each one, recall the conversation and decide if there was a potentially valuable connection for either yourself or someone else. If you promised to send a person a link to a Web site or an article to read, follow through with your promise. In some cases, you'll want to follow up by phone; otherwise, an email will do. For a connection that looks promising, an email suggesting a lunch meeting would be appropriate. Be sure to remind the person where you met and what you think the connection is: "We met at the Bay Area Association for Behavior Analysis on Tuesday night, and I am hoping we can continue our discussion of . . ."

Social Networking

Perhaps the most common form of networking today is the virtual kind. This is where you meet someone online, and then follow up via instant messaging, text messaging, or other online systems. If you get a response, you can follow up with the person and start a conversation that might lead somewhere. Some business networking apps include LinkedIn, Facebook Groups, Shapr, and Bizzabo.[3] On these apps you can create a network for your organization and invite your colleagues or anyone with similar interests to join. Again, we are talking about professional interests here, such as interacting with other behavior analysts who work with preschool children with autism as opposed to social and dating sites. Most of the recommendations for face-to-face networking described earlier apply to this form, i.e., you need to express an interest in the other professionals on the site, come across as sincere and authentic, and be prepared to follow up with anyone who would appear to be a professional match.

YOUNG PROFESSIONAL (3–5 YEARS)

Having made it through your first two years as a behavior analyst, the next three will be much easier. Networking will become second nature and you will be able to size people up more quickly and with more confidence. By now there are probably half a dozen or more serious contacts that you have made that helped you resolve issues at work or think through an ethics problem since they have become trusted colleagues. In the same vein, at least that many have benefited from your connection in finding jobs, recruiting staff, and perhaps entering a business venture together. Along with your experience in networking comes the confidence to model this strategy for your direct reports (RBTs, trainees, BCaBAs, etc.) when you attend conferences or social gatherings with other behavior analysts.

MID-CAREER (6–10 YEARS)

Moving into mid-career as a seasoned behavior analyst with a well-established system, most of your networking will likely be with other civic organizations who can support yours or where you can become mutually engaged in promoting both business and humanitarian causes in your community. The value-added in expanding your network includes increased exposure to your company's expertise and enhancing the opportunities to meet other healthcare professionals as your company expands its consumer base. Sponsoring local fundraising campaigns and supporting job fairs is a way of giving back to the community as well as supporting worthy causes.

SENIOR BEHAVIOR ANALYST

As a professional with over a decade of experience, you will likely be at the top of your organization or business and be involved in management decisions on a regular basis. This will require you to network with Directors and CEOs from other companies as well as attorneys, CPAs, and MDs, as well as your counterparts in other behavioral organizations. Big issues such as licensing and accreditation as well as state legislative matters that affect your company and the profession of behavior analysis will take up much of your time and applying your networking skills honed over many years will be a centerpiece of your repertoire. Being able to call on friends and colleagues to help with important issues and activities is made possible because you maintained a network of professional contacts over the years.

SUMMARY

This chapter describes networking, which is an essential practice for all behavior analysts. Networking is most important for those new graduates who are taking on their first jobs. Networking basically involves meeting new people either in person or online, making a good impression, learning about their leisure activities and career goals, and then maintaining that relationship over time if there are strong mutual interests. Networking can help behavior analysts find their first (or new) jobs, and it can help build professional relationships in current jobs.

NOTES

1 www.davedelaney.me
2 www.apollotechnical.com/networking-statistics/
3 https://krisp.ai/blog/best-networking-apps/

FOR FURTHER READING

Darling, D. C. (2003). *The networking survival guide: Get the success you want by tapping into the people you know*. New York: McGraw-Hill.

Pollard, M. (2021). *The introvert's edge to networking: Work the room, leverage social media, develop powerful connections*. New York: HarperCollins Leadership.

Stonehouse, R. A. (2019). *Power networking for shy people: How to network like a pro*. Amazon: Live for Excellence Productions.

19

Learn to Deal With Stress: A Behavioral Approach

Stress is the harmful physical and emotional responses that occur when the requirements of the job do not match the capabilities, resources, or needs of the worker.

—National Institute for Occupational Safety and Health Administration (1999)

WHAT IS STRESS?

Behavior analysts are particularly prone to stress by the very nature of their work. They often supervise new staff who have little experience, manage a caseload of direct treatment clients, conduct assessments, and write behavior plans. They may be on-call 24 hours at a time, and they chair and attend many meetings. Too many most will say. Adding to the stress there are client families that frequently complain, want to change schedules and behavior plans overnight, and there is an unbelievable amount of turnover in the therapists that they supervise. Driving across town or from one county to another to reach clients who live in remote areas can add further stress to a behavior analyst with an already hectic schedule. Enduring traffic delays or receiving urgent cell phone calls

DOI: 10.4324/9781003265573-23

while you are negotiating a detour can turn the commute from one in-home client to the next into a nightmare. Parents often have an expectation that behavior change will come quickly, and they may act disappointed if little Adam is not cured of his hyperactivity, aggressiveness, or slow learning in just a few sessions. Likewise, clinical directors or owners may expect you to handle "just one more client" and assure you, "It is very much appreciated, you'll see. I'll make this up to you. Just help me out of this jam."

Here is a good example of the current situation from a BCBA writing to the ABA Ethics Hotline (printed with permission):

> I have been at my current job for about 2.5 years. It was acquired by a larger company almost six months ago. Shortly after that, Medicaid rules changed, which significantly increased the amount of paperwork required. After the acquisition I communicated with the new CEO about our caseloads and that we had too much on us, particularly since we were also being told to fill in for therapists who had quit or were out sick. The business is both a combined private day school and therapy center, so we were unable to cancel school clients due to staffing agreed to in the school contracts. Most of our insurance clients are after school. We ended up working 20–30 hours a week direct with clients with no decrease in our supervisory caseload. At this point, I was juggling home duties in addition to working a minimum of 50 hours a week due to the demands of my position. I communicated this incredible workload pressure multiple times to the CEO.
>
> I finally hit a burnout point a little over two months ago, crying and having panic attacks at work on almost a daily basis. I've been in the field as a BCBA for nearly 20 years and I've never felt so incompetent in terms of being behind in my paperwork and programming. I kept asking for help, but they just kept telling me they were trying to hire RBTs, and it would get better. It hasn't. A friend I confided in connected me with a smaller company with better work-life policies and I decided to leave, giving 45-days' notice. The VP tried to retain me, but I told her why I was leaving and that I was moving to a company that will compensate me at the same level with only 30 hours a week—this is what I need for my family.

I've worked as hard as I can during my notice period, but we still have the same staffing issues. My last day is Thursday. At the end of last week, the VP gave me a list of all the paperwork I'm behind on. I'm trying to get it done but I know it's not possible in the time I have left. I want to do the right thing for my clients, but I'm not a superhero. I'm just a burnt-out BCBA.

These standard stress-management approaches do not deal with the *cause* of stress. A contrasting approach is to promote *organizational change* as a solution.

COMMON SYMPTOMS, STANDARD SOLUTIONS

A little stress is not a bad thing, it can sharpen your focus and give you an adrenaline boost in an emergency. Prolonged work-related stress, however, can cause headaches, chest pain, shortness of breath, stomach aches, tiredness, and sleep problems. This in turn may cause anxiety, irritability, mood swings, resentment, and burnout as in the example cited above. The effects on behavior can include skipping meals, overeating, angry outbursts, crying, excessive alcohol consumption, and produce decreased productivity, and spotty work performance. Traditional solutions to life stressors include exercising, relaxing, getting lots of sleep, and in some cases going to counseling or seeing a psychotherapist.[1] One popular non-behavioral approach is to focus on self-care (Fiebig, Gould, Ming, & Watson, 2020), which emphasizes "tools and practices" (p. 559) that the person can use to promote "resilience in the face of practical challenges." Such stress-management approaches do not deal with the *cause* of stress or anxiety, but rather seem to suggest that the person should learn to adapt to an environment that is clearly flawed in terms of "practical challenges" which

The foundation of stress prevention is built on a healthy diet, eight hours of sleep, and vigorous exercise at least three times per week.

are patently unreasonable. A contrasting much more behavioral approach is to promote *environmental change* as a solution.[2] This involves analyzing the stressful factors in a work environment such as excessive workload or assignments outside your scope of competence and modifying your environment to reduce the stress. A behavioral approach to dealing with stress would involve concepts with which we are familiar such as motivational operations, antecedent stimuli, response cost, or contingencies of reinforcement and that still meet the requirements set by Baer, Wolf, and Risley (1968) rather than cognitive approaches like "mindfulness" (Neff & Dahm, 2015).

In addition, you will want to consider the Big Three Factors[3] that if properly balanced can mitigate chronic stress: proper diet, adequate sleep, and sufficient exercise. It can easily happen that you are working so much and so intensely that you are not taking care of your physical health. Living on fried, greasy fast food, gulping down energy drinks, getting only five hours of sleep each night; and engaging in virtually no exercise are a prescription for an emotional or physical breakdown. The foundation of stress prevention is built on a healthy diet, eight hours of sleep, and vigorous exercise at least three times per week. If you don't have this regime in place, consider improving all three to help you deal with other stressors in your life.

FRESH OUT OF GRAD SCHOOL, FIRST JOB

As an enthusiastic new behavior analyst, depending on where you are working for your first job, you may soon realize that you are experiencing the signs of stress. From a behavioral perspective, the organizational change approach makes much more sense than taking up "choiceless awareness meditation," listening to nature sound CDs as you drive down the road or taking hatha yoga classes on Thursday night. If you are overwhelmed by the caseload you have been assigned, find that you are inhaling Reese's Pieces by the handful, and are constantly on the lookout for another "Happy Hour 4:00 till 8:00" sign, taking a Pilates class is not the right solution for you. Pilates and other forms of exercise have clear benefits and will make you strong and fit, but exercise alone will not fix your stress. You must deal with the actual cause. How did you come to have this caseload anyway? Was it a failure to say "no" at just the right time? Are you having difficulty closing out cases? Do you need some help with a difficult client but don't know whom to talk to?

> Perhaps one of the less often considered but surely important ways to reduce stress is to analyze the nature of the work you are doing to determine if it is part of the cause.

So, what can you do to better manage your life? For starters, we recommend opening with a review of the tips in Chapter 16 on time management. Some of your stress may result from not having a reasonable daily and weekly plan that allows you to efficiently get from one clinic or school to the next. If you become stressed because of traffic congestion on your daily commute, look at your schedule to determine if there is a more efficient way to get from A to B to C. Perhaps some of your clients would be willing to change their standing appointments; this might allow you to avoid the morning rush. If some of your stress is related to your always being late, take a close look at factors that could be causing the lateness. One colleague had this frustration and found that he had to take the blame for not informing his clients that he had to be out the door at a fixed time. He was thinking that it was rude to cut off a conversation in mid-sentence. By informing these clients at the beginning of his necessary departure time, he was able to prompt them with, "Okay, Mrs. Rudd. I have only 5 minutes before I must leave." By exercising a combination of assertiveness, time management, and personal communications skills, he was able to leave on time and avoid speeding through traffic lights to get to his next appointment.

External Stressors

Perhaps one of the less often considered but surely important ways to reduce stress is to analyze the nature of the work you are doing to determine if it is part of the cause. There was probably a point early in your present job where you felt that you had everything under control. You understood your client's problem, you had cooperation wfrom your stakeholders, your behavior program was getting good results, and you got recognition and a bonus from the CEO. Life was good. Then somehow everything got out of control. What exactly happened? Once you have been on the job long enough, did you agree to supervise two new RBTs, only to discover that they required a lot of handholding? Or was it the case of the single mother with the autistic child who was progressing so nicely and then somehow hit a plateau that is causing stress? This child's mother started to ask questions about applied behavior analysis. She was reading articles about special diets and wondering if maybe applied behavior analysis wasn't the solution after all. Picky, picky, picky. It was nerve-racking; she just wouldn't be satisfied with what you told her and wanted to talk to the clinical director. And then your supervisor took the mom's side and started questioning your program plan. Now *that* can make a person jumpy.

And remember when your roommate suddenly decided to leave town, and you got stuck with the whole month's rent until the lease ran out? This is when you started wearing the T-shirt that said, "**STRESS**: *The confusion created when one's mind overrides the body's basic desire to choke the living daylights out of someone who desperately deserves it.*"[4] Thanks to your roommate who bailed on you with no notice, you had to take on three extra cases to make up the difference in rent money: "I'm young and I don't have a partner right now so I can do 50 hours a week . . . at least until I find a roommate."

What To Do About Stress: A Behavioral Approach

Much of the traditional literature and advice on the internet has to do with identifying the signs of stress and taking steps to manage the symptoms. Behavior analysts who trust their ability to understand human behavior, including their own, are likely to reject this strategy in favor of a more comfortable, familiar behavioral approach. After all, if a client came to you with all these symptoms, wouldn't you start with pinpointing the behaviors and conducting a functional analysis?

Step 1: Pinpoint the Stressful Emotions, Feelings, and Behaviors

As with any situation you would encounter at work, you know the first thing you must do is pinpoint the behavior or result that is causing the problem. Is it actually physical? Chest pains, shortness of breath, anxiety? If so, a medical check-up by your family physician is certainly called for. What about behaviors that you've adopted that look like they could cause trouble down the line: overeating, crying spells, or decreased productivity? You know how to make lists and data sheets, so start with this. Chart your symptoms (both behavioral and physical) to determine the frequency and make a column for possible antecedents. You should note the time of day as well as coincidental events. For example, if your anxiety goes up around 3:00 p.m. on some days but not others, look at your appointment book or iCal and see what was going on leading up to 3:00. Is it racing through traffic or dealing with your family that appears to be sabotaging your own healthy living treatment plan? Does this happen only on days when you were up late the night before and didn't get enough sleep? You can analyze your data by using a standard ABC analysis (antecedent—behavior—consequence) with the addition of "Setting Event" as a broad category of rather vague issues that might set the occasion for a range of unpleasant experiences during the following day (see Figure 19.1).

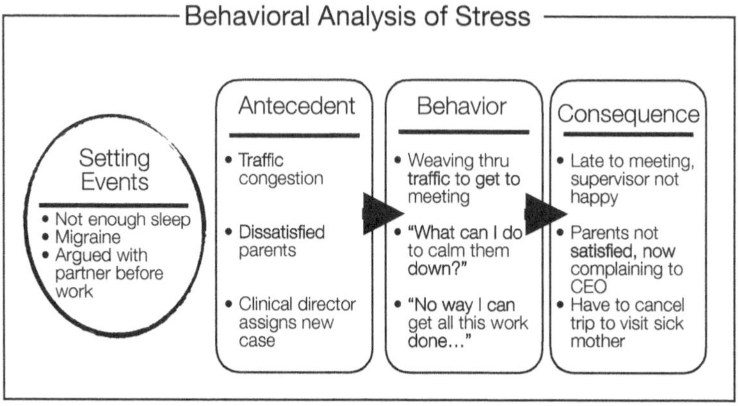

Figure 19.1 Examples of setting events and antecedents that cause stress.

Step 2: Perform a Functional Analysis

This is going to be tricky because you are essentially experimenting with yourself. Be objective about this, starting with recording instances of problematic behavior and troublesome emotional states. A scatter plot graph that you fill in each time you experience anxiety, chest pains, or food cravings might look like the one in Figure 19.2. These are color-coded to show black for chest pains, dark gray for anxiety, and light gray for food cravings. Next, it is necessary to look back through your daily planner to identify which events were associated with these symptoms of stress in your life.

To determine if your hypothesis is correct and you have in fact identified the controlling variable, you will need to make a temporary change in your schedule or sequence of events. Consulting on three intense client cases back-to-back without a break may be just too much or racing across town for a supervision meeting with no time to review your notes may be too much. By changing your schedule and honestly and objectively recording the results, you should be able to isolate the factors that are causing stress in your life. Some variables will be difficult to manipulate, especially if they occur infrequently, such as too little sleep or an argument

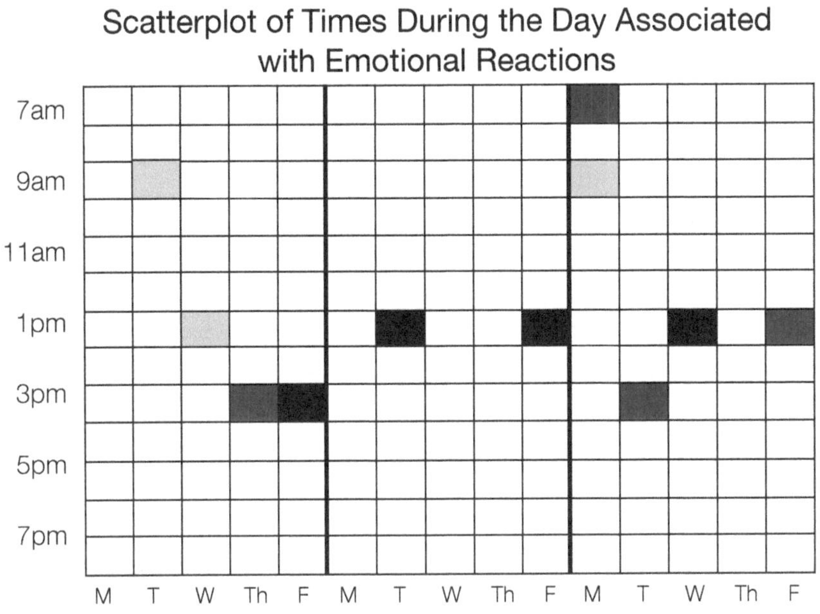

Figure 19.2 Scatter plot graph of times of day that cause an emotional reaction.
Note: Black is for chest pains, dark gray is for anxiety, and light gray is for food cravings.

with your spouse or partner. Are you staying up late because you drank too much coffee at dinner, or because you have a habit of watching late-night television shows every night, or because you possibly have a disturbed sleep pattern (sleep apnea)? If the problem is the latter, your physician should be able to run the necessary tests to isolate the medical condition. If your sleep problems are related to your getting wound up when you watch late-night television, it may be time for you to invest in a recording device so you can watch your favorite late-night shows at an earlier time. This is the sort of functional analysis you would perform when a client expressed concern about anxiety or poor performance. You owe it to yourself to apply what you know to solve your own personal problems.

One serious cause of stress and anxiety is a workload increase beyond what is humanly possible for behavior analysts who feel

> You owe it to yourself to apply what you know to solve your own personal problems.

obligated to follow the BACB Ethics Code. Many administrators and Clinical Directors feel that in their need to increase the bottom line they must increase client billable hours, RBT direct hours, and supervisor caseloads. You don't have to be Sherlock Holmes to establish that this sort of constant pressure is the cause of much fear and anxiety. The answer is simple but comes with considerable risk. When the clinical director comes to you with two big file folders and says, "Guess what I have for you?" the only response that will save you is, "I'm sorry I cannot take on any more clients." The risk is that you might be let go, but you do have leverage since there are far more jobs than there are behavior analysts available. In anticipation of this situation, always make sure when you are being interviewed to ask about your caseload and other expectations. This is the time to negotiate this critical employment factor. Then make sure you have this in writing in your contract.

Step 3: Develop a Short-Term Intervention

Depending on what you discover from your functional analysis, it may be possible to work out a short-term solution that will provide some relief while you work on a long-term solution. For example, if you discover that your stress level goes down during the day when you get more sleep the night before, a quick fix might just be a matter of better time management and some discipline regarding television shows or late-night phone conversations with friends and relatives. The same goes for variables that produce stress during the day. Being resolute with your supervisor and making it clear that when you finish these three overload cases, you will *not* pick up any more could go a long way toward relieving your stressful week. Likewise, when working with a client who appears to be dissatisfied with your services and is about to complain to your boss, consult with your supervisor before the client does (you'll feel tremendous relief). Your supervisor might provide the resources to help you with the client or decide that it is time to transfer this client to another behavioral consultant.

Step 4: Develop and Adopt a Long-Term Plan

Your long-term plan, which you might be working on to bring to fruition in six months or longer, could involve some rather major changes in your life:

- separating from the argumentative significant other,
- changing jobs,
- working for a smaller company,
- moving to a rural area where the living is less hectic,
- setting up your own private practice one you have the experience needed, work for yourself, set your own hours (this might be a 2-year goal), and
- moving out of a noisy apartment into your own condo or home.

These are all examples of ways to relieve stress that involve a good deal of planning and possibly some hardship and additional stress in the short term.

YOUNG PROFESSIONAL (3–5 YEARS)

If you have made it this far in your career, you have probably figured out a way to manage your work so that it fits comfortably with your lifestyle. This history of understanding what is doable in the time allowed and pushing back on everything else has likely given you room to breathe and hopefully made you a better colleague and supervisor. With this experience, you are now able to work with supervisees to assure that you don't put unreasonable demands on them and that you always attend to their feedback. You can also teach supervisees to analyze the stressful elements in their work and personal situations (refer them to Figures 19.1 and

19.2 in this chapter) and to work toward eliminating or modifying them. If you have an HR department, you can ask them to conduct regular independent surveys to make sure that all employees feel they are listened to and that they have input.

MID-CAREER (6–10 YEARS)

Making it to mid-career clearly shows that you have what it takes to balance your work and the rest of your life. Now you may be able to help set company policy related to working conditions for all behavior analysts in the firm. While a completely stress-free environment is probably not possible, understanding the factors that cause stress and implementing company-wide measures to eliminate or at least mitigate those factors is a worthy endeavor.

SENIOR BEHAVIOR ANALYST

Once you have reached this status, you will clearly be able to influence the culture of your business or organization. You can advance the position that they will not institute policies and procedures that directly or indirectly affect the work-related stress of employees. Traditional companies that are not behavioral will routinely attempt to improve the bottom line by increasing caseloads, thinning out supervision, and admitting challenging clients when they do not have the trained staff to accommodate their needs. As a behavior analyst and leader in the organization who is interested in maintaining a stable, happy, efficient, and productive workforce, you should be able to detect those factors that are guaranteed to increase stress and work to eliminate them.

SUMMARY

This chapter described a behaviorally oriented approach to stress in the workplace. Behavior analysts are particularly prone to stress by the very nature of their work. They often supervise new staff who have little experience, manage a caseload of direct treatment clients, conduct assessments, write behavior plans, and more, much more each week. Sadly, we have a burnout phenomenon on our hands that can be laid at the feet of the companies where behavior analysts are employed. Symptoms of stress include headaches, chest pain, shortness of breath, stomach aches, tiredness, and sleep problems. These may in turn cause anxiety, irritability, mood swings, resentment, decreased productivity, and spotty work performance. Stress can be mitigated to a certain extent through proper diet, adequate sleep, and sufficient exercise. Reducing or eliminating stressful contingencies can be done in four steps, and behavior analysts owe it to themselves to manage their own stress.

NOTES

1 See the Mayo Clinic Web site: mayoclinic.com/health/stress-symptoms.
2 See cdc.gov/niosh/stresswk.html
3 www.cdc.gov/violenceprevention/about/copingwith-stresstips.html
4 https://boinc.berkeley.edu/dev/forum_thread.php?id=11551

REFERENCES

Baer, D. M., Wolf, M. M., & Risley, T. R. (1968). Some current dimensions of applied behavior analysis. *Journal of Applied Behavior Analysis*, *1*, 91–97.

Fiebig, J. H., Gould, E. R., Ming, S., & Watson, R. A. (2020). An invitation to act on the value of self-care: Being a whole person in all that you do. *Behavior Analysis in Practice*, *13*, 559–567.

National Institute for Occupational Safety and Health Administration. (1999). www.cdc.gov/niosh/stresswk.html. Publication No. 99–101.

Neff, K. D., & Dahm, K. A. (2015). Self-compassion: What it is, what it does, and how it relates to mindfulness. In B. D. Ostafin, M. D. Robinson, & B. P. Meier (Eds.), *Handbook of mindfulness and self-regulation* (pp. 121–137). New York: Springer.

20

Public Speaking

Speech is power: speech is to persuade, to convert, to compel.

—Ralph Waldo Emerson

FRESH OUT OF GRAD SCHOOL, FIRST JOB

It is estimated that glossophobia (the fear of public speaking) affects 75% of the population.[1] Most people simply cannot imagine themselves standing in front of a large audience of strangers and giving a talk. Phobic public speakers begin to think of every disaster that might happen during a presentation, "What if they don't like me? What if I choke up and forget what I'm supposed to say? What if the projector doesn't work? What if they ask me a question, and I don't know the answer?" This line of negative thinking is common for beginning public speakers. Once you are practiced and experienced, you might have mild nervousness before a big talk, but the intense panic will be gone. For experienced, confident speakers who have given talks and would like to brush up on their skills, we have some suggestions that will help you catch the next wave in technology and public speaking theory so you can become a great public speaker.

It is estimated that glossophobia (fear of public speaking) affects 75% of the population.

DOI: 10.4324/9781003265573-24

Most graduate students will not have taken a public speaking course during their 2–4 years in their master's or PhD programs, and yet a great deal of the job of a behavior analyst involves just that; speaking to families and colleagues in meetings large and small as well as presenting a paper or giving a CE workshop. If you are using slides, you will want to take care to respect the confidentiality of your clients by not using photos of them where their faces are shown. Our advice is to take every opportunity to participate in "small talks" as they will be great practice for later and lay the foundation for giving larger talks.

Giving presentations to civic organizations or healthcare groups is probably the best way to spread the word about behavior analysis and as a person who is new to the field, you may be called on to do this on behalf of your company. These will likely be informal talks and you may be provided with the text and slide deck by the HR or marketing department. Some new companies have an outreach strategy to educate physicians about ABA and these will be "Lunch and Learn" sessions in their offices. The goal is to let the community know about your company, give them a glimpse of what behavior analysis is and answer any questions they might have.

With practice and training, you'll get to the point where you can address a larger audience who will sense your caring and sincerity, your enthusiasm for behavior analysis will come through loud and clear, and you'll soon be able to resolve any misconceptions that others have about our field.

As a general plan related to your public speaking progress, as a "Fresh Out of Grad School" behavior analyst, think of starting with presentations for your colleagues in your company (e.g., at meetings), then progressing to presentations for the local community, and finally moving on to giving presentations at the state level followed by public speaking at national (and possibly international) meetings.

How to Get Started

It is not a bad idea to start collecting and reading some recent books on public speaking (Acker, 2021; Anderson, 2017; Blesenbach, 2018). When you attend conferences, pay special attention to the best ABA speakers there, e.g., Dr. Pat Friman, Lorrie Unumb, Shawn Cappell, Dr. Greg Hanley, and Dr. Bridget Taylor to see if you can pick up some tips.

If you have given small talks that have gone well but the idea of presenting in front of a crowd makes you tremble with fear (possible glossophobia), you can approach this as you would any fear by using *in vivo* desensitization. Desensitization works by gradual exposure to the fear-producing stimulus so that the anxiety gradually goes on extinction. How long this takes depends on how often you practice, and it will vary from one person to the next. If it looks like you are not making any progress by yourself, you might consider finding a behavior therapist to help you. It is worth it to do whatever it takes to overcome your fear. To maximize your effectiveness as a behavior analyst, you need to push yourself to the point where you can address most any audience on short notice and tell your story with confidence and enthusiasm.

Standard Techniques for Public Speaking

Preparing Your Talk

There are two parts to every talk: (a) the *content* (this is your message) and (b) the *delivery*. Most people worry most about the delivery and what they are going to do with their hands, how they are going to project their voice, and how they will move around the room or the stage. But it is impossible to be a great public speaker without having a compelling message to deliver. You need to begin with a good story (Simmons, 2019) that you feel comfortable and excited about telling. This should be a story you know so well you don't need a script to tell it.

Step 1: Identify the Key Points of Your Talk You won't have time to cover an endless number of details, so start by outlining your presentation to determine what is reasonable to cover in the time allotted. Most speakers attempt to include too much content, and then they feel rushed to cover it all. Big mistake. You'll be better off if you pare down your talk to about half a dozen important points in a 30-minute talk. Once you have your key points, determine the order in which they will be presented. It is very helpful to think in terms of a "story arc" with a beginning, middle, and end as shown in Figure 20.1. For behavior analysts, these will often include a problem or challenge you came upon or were given, followed by an intense inquiry and some developmental research possibly using a creative functional analysis. The middle of your talk will convey in vivid terms the solution that you arrived at after much work and deliberation; then as you coast to the end you will be able to present the outcome and the benefit to the client(s), the school, or society at large.

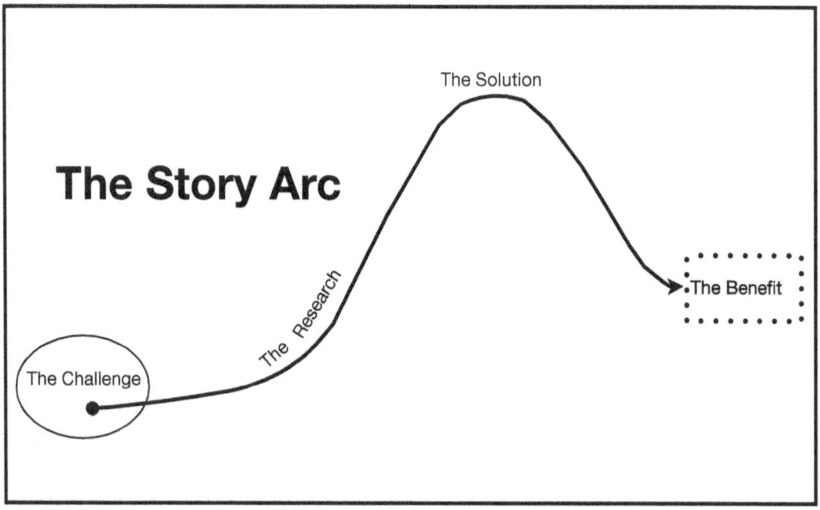

Figure 20.1 This figure shows the standard story arc for a behavior analysis presentation.

Step 2: Finding the Hook Another tip for developing the perfect presentation is to start with the following mandate: "I need to give my audience a reason to listen to me. Why should they care?" This is the question a great speaker will answer within the first 90 seconds of a presentation. You should start with a *hook* to get your audience interested. A hook can be a question to the audience such as, "How many of you have had to endure someone sitting next to you talking loudly on his cell phone?", a humorous story, a well-chosen quote, some dramatic statistic, or a "look ahead" that will result in your audience wanting to hear more. An example of a beginning that will cause the audience to think, "What happened next?" is the following introduction used by one behavior analyst consultant. "Little 7-year-old Maria stumbled to her desk, pulled out her notebook, and wrote 'Help Me' in large letters with a stubby crayon. Then she put her head down and began sobbing." This was a well-chosen, dramatic beginning for a presentation given to school officials. This single anecdote had everyone in the room paying close attention to the speaker, who was giving a talk on individualized education programs that could have otherwise been routine and boring.

Step 3: Presenting the Content Once you have the attention of the audience, you can proceed to the content of your presentation. This will be the bulk of the presentation, although you must resist the urge to put too much material into this middle section. Your goal in the content section of the talk is to acquaint the audience members with the topic, show them how it is relevant, and motivate them to learn more. Rather than have slide after slide of bullet points that you read aloud, you will want to focus on the highlights as a progression.[2] Make sure the material is presented in an organized fashion and you adequately explain the concepts without burying the audience in tiny details.

Step 4: End With a BANG! For the ending of your presentation, come back to the teaser and finish that story or provide one final anecdote that will give your talk a memorable ending. This could be a dramatic photo on the screen that tells a story in and of itself, a final humorous anecdote, or a quote that wraps up the essence of your talk. There seems to be a *primacy* effect and a *recency* effect (Gelb, 2020, pp. 71–72) with audiences. If people are asked later about the talk, they are more likely to remember the beginning and the end rather than the middle. This is another good reason to present just a few key points and follow them up with a handout that you distribute at the end of your talk.

> It is your prerogative to ask for changes to make certain the room suits *your* needs and requirements.

Practice Your Delivery

The first recommendation for a great delivery is practice, practice, practice. This comes from countless books on public speaking and Toastmasters International,[3] the leading organization in the United States that teaches and promotes good public speaking. Practice in front of a mirror, practice with a friend, and finally, if possible, practice in the room where you will be speaking. Taping your practice talks and reviewing them in the privacy of your office will enable you to objectively analyze how your presentation looks from the audience's side. Videotapes will show you if your body language was stiff and might provide the feedback you need to try a different style of presenting, such as stepping away from the podium, using a wireless mic, or actually walking right up the center aisle and around the audience where you can see people up close and talk directly to them. You will need a wireless remote if you are going to go mobile and show slides at the same time, but this can be a powerful demonstration that you know your material and is worth the extra time it takes to prepare and organize a set-up like this.

The second recommended practice for a successful presentation, right after cleaning out your pockets, of course, is to relax. This might seem very difficult given the stress associated with talking to large crowds, but it works. Just before you go on stage, and while you are out of sight, take several deep breaths. Remember that you are having a conversation about a topic that you know well and that you are here just to tell your story. These people wouldn't have invited you if they didn't want to hear your story. You'll be fine.

> **Great slide presentations contain appropriate content, arranged in the most efficient, graceful manner without superfluous decoration.**

The final recommendation for a good delivery is to make sure that you are in your conversational mode and that you feel comfortable changing your tone of voice, from soft to loud and back, and using pauses for effect. If you have looked at yourself on tape and know that you have a tendency toward a monotone voice, absolutely make sure that you avoid this voice like you would avoid a giant pothole in front of your house. In a normal conversation with people, you will laugh, make jokes, and tell stories. All this is perfectly acceptable in your presentations as long as you keep it clean, and the jokes and stories are relevant to your message. At a recent conference in front of 500 people, one of the invited speakers started his talk like this: "I've been told that I'm a very dry speaker and that I should start my talk with a joke. Okay, so here's the joke . . ." Unfortunately, the joke wasn't funny, it wasn't related to the topic, and no one laughed. He had a hard time recovering, and even though he was a recognized expert in his field, he surely did not have the impact he wanted. To his credit, he had a 20-page handout with all the key points and references for people to pick up at the podium when the talk was over.

Avoid Death by PowerPoint There is currently a counterrevolution going on against standard, ubiquitous, *boring*, PowerPoint-type presentations. Described as a reaction to "death by PowerPoint," this movement is out to revolutionize presentations by starting over with a new goal. Rather than asking, "How much text can I squeeze onto a page?" the group of creative designers leading the new wave proposed, "Great slide presentations contain appropriate content, arranged in the most efficient, graceful manner without superfluous decoration. The presentation is simple, balanced, and beautiful" (Reynolds, 2019, p. 25). Reynolds went on to say:

> Live talks enhanced by multimedia are about storytelling and have more in common with the art of documentary film than the reading of a paper document. Live talks today must tell a story enhanced by imagery and other forms of appropriate multimedia. (p. 25)

Try Presentation Zen This new approach, called *Presentation Zen* by Reynolds (2019), takes its meaning from clean and simple Japanese designs for products. In fact, Reynolds credits an experience he had many years ago when he was eating lunch out of a *bento* (a type of Japanese lunch box) in a Tokyo train station. He happened to see a businessman flipping through page after page of PowerPoint slides printed two to a page. They were crammed with headers and bullet points, which contrasted with his *bento*, which was "beautifully efficient, well-designed . . . nothing superfluous" (Reynolds, 2019, p. 6). Reynolds concluded that technical presentations could be made simple and beautiful as well. Reynolds's book is a must-read for anyone assigned to give a presentation or who wants to improve her public speaking. The basic concepts include having a minimalist approach to text, putting very few words on a slide, and not using lists of bullet points (gasp!). Instead, use captivating photos or compelling graphics to tell your story. For a 20-minute talk, no more than 20 slides are recommended. To see an example of simple, elegant presentations, go to www.ted.com.

YOUNG PROFESSIONAL (3–5 YEARS)

Once you have settled into your new job and have given a few dozen small talks in your community you may be ready to take it to a larger stage by giving a presentation at a state conference.

This will require quite a bit more of organizing your material and practicing sufficiently to keep it interesting for the standard 50 minutes that are allotted.

MID-CAREER (6–10 YEARS)

At mid-career with lots of speaking experience you are probably ready for The Big Show which is a national conference such as the annual meeting of the Association for Behavior Analysis International held every year around Memorial Day. This conference draws upwards of 5,000 behavior analysts from all over the world including some of the best speakers. You have probably been attending this conference for a few years and have some idea of what is involved in these presentations. Even though it is an international conference, there is still room for talks that are presented in a smaller room so that you can have some experience on a smaller scale before you submit a paper that might be assigned to a room that will seat 1,000 attendees. If you have a chance to catch a talk by Dr. Pat Friman, you will see him demonstrate how he uses his 15-step method of effective public speaking (Friman, 2014).

SENIOR BEHAVIOR ANALYST

At this point in your career, and with many, many conferences, and presentations behind you, you may be invited to give a big presentation on the topic on which you are considered an expert. At ABAI, they have categories of big talks that are called Tutorials, Invited Presenter, and the B.F. Skinner Lecture Series. These represent a speaker's accumulated knowledge and experience in their area of expertise. Expectations are very high for these talks both in terms of content and any visuals that accompany them. Speakers at this level will often have graphic artists at their companies put together the slide shows which may include not only striking visuals but may also be accompanied by video clips and animations.

SUMMARY

This chapter described the importance of public speaking as a necessary part of every behavior analyst's repertoire. Many people have a fear of public speaking (glossophobia). This fear can inhibit a behavior analyst's ability to convey to clients, colleagues, and community audiences the breadth and scope of our field. The best way to acquire public speaking skills is to start small by speaking up at meetings and volunteering to present at intimate gatherings and in-house training sessions. Four primary steps are depicted as necessary for giving a good talk. These include identifying your key points, finding the "hook" to get audiences interested, effectively presenting the content, and ending with a bang. Additional essentials are how to set up your room, test your equipment, and meet your audience just prior to your talk. Knowing how to present an impressive slide show and using music to enhance your presentation will mark you as an engaging, proficient speaker.

NOTES

1 www.psycom.net/glossophobia-fear-of-public-speaking
2 If your talk has a lot of content, this is best handled with a handout. Make this available at the end of the presentation.
3 Go to www.toastmasters.org for a complete set of recommendations on public speaking and a way to find a group near you.

FOR FURTHER READING

Duarte, N. (2008). *DataStory: Explain data and inspire action through story*. Oakton, VA: Ideapress Publishing.

Duarte, N. (2008). *Slide:ology: The art and science of creating great presentations*. Sebastopol, CA: O'Reilly Media.

Gallo, C. (2010). *The presentation secrets of Steve Jobs*. New York: McGraw-Hill.

REFERENCES

Acker, M. (2021). *Speak with no fear: Go from a nervous, nauseated, and sweaty speaker to an excited, energized, and passionate presenter* (2nd ed.). Daphne, AL: Advantage Publishing Group.

Anderson, C. (2017). *Ted talks: The official TED guide to public speaking* (repr. ed.). New York: Harper Business.
Blesenbach, R. (2018). *Unleash the power of storytelling: Win hearts, change minds, get results*. Evanston, IL: Eastlawn Media.
Friman, P. C. (2014). Behavior analysts to the front! A 15-step tutorial on public speaking. *The Behavior Analyst, 37*, 109–118.
Gelb, M. J. (2020). *Mastering the art of public speaking: 8 secrets to transform fear and supercharge your career*. Novato, CA: New World Library.
Reynolds, G. (2019). *Presentationzen: Simple ideas on presentation design and delivery*. Berkeley, CA: New Riders.
Simmons, A. (2019). *The story factor: Inspiration, influence, and persuasion through the art of storytelling*. Cambridge, MA: Basic Books.
www.Ted.com (Technology, Entertainment, Design).

Unit

Five

Advanced Skills

A CEO speaking to his Clinical Director . . .

> Well, I had my quarterly meeting with the BCBAs yesterday. We talked about insurance and billing and other routine issues. The one thing that got me unsettled was when the behavioral staff started talking about the growing trend toward off-the-shelf downloadable behavior programs for behavior problems and language training. I am not happy with this way of thinking, and I wanted to bring it up with you. My granddaughter has ASD and if she was one of our clients, I would want her to receive individualized treatment. I think we need some creative thinking here, and some new ideas on how to design custom-made therapy methods that fit each family's needs and that will be easily adopted into their daily lives. If our behavioral staff wants to be more efficient, they need to be curious and look for other solutions. Can you check into this and get back to me?

DOI: 10.4324/9781003265573-25

21

Creative Problem-Solving and Troubleshooting

Life is trying things to see if they work.

—Ray Bradbury

FRESH OUT OF GRAD SCHOOL, FIRST JOB

Our clients and stakeholders would have no need for a behavior analyst if they could deal with their problems themselves. They have no doubt tried all the obvious solutions based on *their* own understanding of human behavior. What most clients need is a creative solution, and they expect us to be experts in developing these. Identifying the behavior problem, finding a way to measure it, conducting an assessment, and writing a behavior program are all the initial steps involved in creative problem-solving. In *Phase 1*, once we develop an evidence-based, functional, ethical, and practical behavior plan and implement it, we are on to the next phase. *Phase 2* is troubleshooting the plan when it breaks down. Most of the training we provide our behavior analysis graduate students is directed at Phase 1 where in classroom and practicum settings, students learn how to pinpoint problem behaviors, measure them precisely, find the cause of behavior problems through observation and functional analysis, and write and implement behavior programs. Although outsiders might consider this a

DOI: 10.4324/9781003265573-26

novel approach, for us it is routine. In most cases we can find the function of the behavior and identify reinforcers; the hard part comes in figuring out how to teach replacement behaviors and change the contingencies in such a way as to modify the behavior without causing harm. Of course, all of this should be done on a timetable that is reasonable for our clients.

Phase 1: Creative Problem-Solving

If an agency or company specializes in treating behavior problems, there is a good chance you will see similar behavior problems on a routine basis. You'll be able to develop your own successful patterns of problem-solving. For self-injurious behavior (SIB), you might look for escape contingencies or automatic reinforcement; for classroom disruptive behaviors, you will probably look to accidental teacher reinforcement, peer attention, and escape from (difficult, uninteresting, inappropriate, ill-suited) academic tasks (often referred to as "Demands"). Occasionally there won't be an apparent solution, and your standard modus operandi will fail you. Now what? Fortunately, we can look to other approaches outside of behavior analysis for some help. In *Why Not?* Nalebuff and Ayres (2006) offered several strategies from an economist and a lawyer who have been helping businesspeople develop creative solutions for years. Perhaps our field could benefit from thinking differently about some of our behavior problems.

Unlimited Resources

One strategy to employ when you are unable to think of a solution is to step back and ask yourself, "What would I do if I had unlimited resources like a university-based lab?" When we can't seem to find the function of a behavior, we might find it helpful to daydream for a moment about having unlimited resources to do a complete experimental functional assessment. If we had a well-equipped laboratory, plenty of graduate assistants, and a computerized data collection system, surely, we could test out enough variables to get to the bottom of the problem. In a setting like this, you could manipulate each variable, scramble the order, replicate conditions, and arrive at a definitive answer. But in the absence of the cold, hard cash, what can you do? One solution is to send your client to a place that does have such facilities. If the behavior is life-threatening, as in the case of self-injury or a severe eating disorder, sometimes special funding sources can be found. Or you could bring someone from a specialized lab like this to your setting and request a consultation to help you create some approximation to well-controlled conditions (Iwata, Dorsey, Slifer, Bauman, & Richman, 1994). You could also consider Wilder, Chen, Atwell, Pritchard, and Weinstein's (2006) work on brief functional analysis and create controlled conditions of very short durations.

Where Else Would It Work?

Another exercise that Nalebuff and Ayres (2006) recommend is to take a solution you thought of for one problem and think about where else it can be applied. This is the classic "solution in search of a problem."

> Tom Coleman and Bill Schlotter, two postal delivery men, were inspired on Halloween night in 1987. They saw a trick-or-treater carrying bright, green-glowing Cyalume light sticks. What else could these light sticks be used for? Have you ever considered glowing candy? If you mount a lollipop on top of one of these sticks, the light would shine through the candy, creating a weird and fun effect. Coleman and Schlotter sold their *Glow Pop* to *Cap Candy*. Their next innovation was an even bigger hit.
>
> (Nalebuff and Ayres; 2006, pp. 31–32)

Flipping It

One final strategy that Nalebuff and Ayres (2006) suggested that seems like it could be useful to behavior analysts who are looking for a creative solution is an exercise called "flipping it." In this exercise, you basically consider what would happen if a standard product or service were reversed or flipped over. Consumers saw this in recent years when creative designers at the H.J. Heinz Company finally figured out a way to help us get the ketchup out of the bottle. They redesigned the container so that it now sits on the table upside down in a squeezable plastic bottle! In behavior analysis, we consider the contingency involving contingent reinforcement to be central to the way that behavior change is engineered. What if we flipped this around so that reinforcers were noncontingent? This has been demonstrated in the research literature and seems to have made headway in clinical and educational applications. If an individual will work hard and undergo a lot of pain to get a reinforcer, why don't we just give it to them and see what happens? We have a concept to explain how this works: the Motivating Operation (MO). By reducing the power of the MO, we greatly reduce the strength of the behavior, perhaps to the point where we could again begin to use the reinforcer contingently to shape an appropriate behavior.

What about other standard operating procedures for behavior change such as when in a classroom we try to train a teacher to give reinforcers contingent on a disruptive student's quiet behavior? What if we prompted the child to reinforce the teacher? Or what about an unruly child who is sent to the office? Instead, what if the child reported to the office first thing in the morning and got her assignment there, and if she completed it, she could visit her classroom for a short time? On one consulting assignment, there was a young man we'll call Marc. He lived in a community residential program, and he wouldn't pull his pants up for anyone or anything. As a part of his program, he lost privileges if he went around without his pants or with his pants down. As a result, he never got to go on any outings. One day, a new bus driver who didn't know about this rule took Marc to the mall with six other clients who were all diagnosed with moderate mental retardation. When the driver and clients got back, the staff rushed the driver and shouted, "What happened?" The driver said, "Nothing. Why?" When told about Marc's program, the bus driver looked stunned and said, "Marc wasn't one bit of a problem. When we got to the mall, he hiked up his pants, and off we went. I didn't even prompt him."

Phase 2: Troubleshooting

In behavior analysis, the fun really begins when your program plan is finally approved. Now it's time to start training all the people involved to play their new roles as *behavior therapists*. Because we work with the model that behavioral interventions are best done in the natural environment by those who live there and work with the clients, this is where we need to look when the program flops. These indigenous individuals know your client well and can often yield the information needed to redesign the key elements. These helpers are indispensable, invaluable, and essential to the behavior-change effort. They can also be unreliable, inconsistent, and sensitive to minor setbacks that are as inevitable as a hurricane in September. We greatly underestimate how much training and support our therapists need, and the first form of troubleshooting involves looking at these partners. Basic troubleshooting involves three steps which are generating a hypothesis about what went wrong, making corrections, and then evaluating them.

As described earlier, most behavior plans have many moving parts, and a lot of things can go wrong. People can forget to provide prompts, they can be inconsistent in the delivery of reinforcers, or they can pair reinforcers with an unpleasant look or a sarcastic comment. Sometimes your chief assistant, a teacher aide, for example, just doesn't show up, and you have no backup—the list goes on and on. In one classroom, we set up a great token economy as a pilot and were prepared to expand it to the entire sixth grade when we discovered that an enterprising student made counterfeit tokens and was selling them on a black market in the cafeteria. In another case, a mom who was trained quite carefully to use backward chaining with her child, starting with shoe tying, gave up after a couple of days and decided her daughter who had a mild disability could just wear flip-flops to school. A gym teacher who was shown how to use a modified time-out procedure to manage disruptive behavior in his class was seen standing over a bench full of middle school youths, berating them for not following instructions to "sit quietly and not talk," while the rest of the class was out of control on the soccer field. Basically, Murphy's Law applies to *all* behavioral interventions: "If anything can go wrong, it will." Behavior analysis is second nature to us, but it may be a foreign language to others. In these examples, troubleshooting led to a different approach to training.

Troubleshooting Tips on Your First Job

Troubleshooting Tip 1 As you are getting started on your first job as a BCBA, you are likely to be involved in training RBTs; make sure to train them to meet a specified criterion (Mager, 1975, 1988; Mager & Pipe, 1984). Design your training to prevent errors. Do not assume that just because you've demonstrated how you want something done and asked, "Any questions?" you are finished. Even if no hands go up when you ask you can bet that someone is confused. Training should follow this order: 1) Describe what you want, 2) give the rationale for it, 3) demonstrate the procedure, 4) have the RBTs/trainees practice the procedure, 5) give immediate feedback, 6) practice some more, 7) give additional positive feedback, and 8) repeat until the trainees are *fluent* with their new routine.

Troubleshooting Tip 2 The first day that your treatment is to start, *be there*. Troubleshooting is only possible if you have seen your intervention implemented. If you let your new intervention start without your being present, you will have to rely on hearsay descriptions, which are guaranteed to be incomplete.

Troubleshooting Tip 3 Always debrief after the first day, and the second day, and the third day. Watch your trainees closely as they describe how they think it went. You will be reading body language to see if they felt comfortable in their new role or perhaps felt ill at ease with the tasks that were assigned to them.

Troubleshooting Tip 4 Measure your outcome. Your behavior plan should be evaluated by the data that are coming in each day. Graph the data every day and be critical of your own work.

Troubleshooting Tip 5 Always have a *Plan B* and be prepared to start over with a new analysis starting with the basic functions of the behavior if your intervention is failing.

YOUNG PROFESSIONAL (3–5 YEARS)

As you gain experience in developing effective behavior-change treatments and interventions with your team of techs and therapists you will likely have more efficient and creative problem-solving strategies that suit your style, match your client caseload, and fit in with your company's policies and procedures. In this period, it will be a good time to reflect on somewhat larger problems and you should look for creative solutions for them as well. At this stage in your career, you may be called on by the administration to help new BCBAs set up their teams to be more effective. Your problem-solving skills will be put to the test to find ways to more quickly train and effectively supervise their RBTs, teach them the "soft skills" necessary to interface successfully with caregivers and teachers, and implement more complex behavior reduction programs. Finding ways of developing empathy, "emotional intelligence," communication skills, and "self-awareness" (Biro, 2020), for example, will require a great deal of problem-solving and some troubleshooting as well.

MID-CAREER (6–10 YEARS)

At mid-career, most behavior analysts are considered professionals who can see the big picture regarding ABA. If you have remained with your original company or were hired to work for a different organization, you will be called on to offer solutions to larger-scale problems. This will be an opportunity to show what you have learned about creative problem-solving. Setting up creative problem-solving workshops for BCBAs and other key staff may be in order if you feel that middle-management stays overloaded in dealing with routine company issues.

With your several-years-experience in troubleshooting individual behavior plans, you may be able to generalize that experience to broader issues. If your company's standard solution to employee morale problems involves a motivational speaker, you could suggest approaching this issue from a troubleshooting perspective. Specifically, after defining "morale"—what if we took random data samples of the relevant behavior or conducted frequent focus groups to discuss possible causes? Could we make mid-course corrections to the way that the work is completed or that feedback is given (or worse, not given)?

SENIOR BEHAVIOR ANALYST

As a person with more than a decade of experience in ABA and who is now possibly part of senior management at a company or association, you will be able to spread the word about the importance of creative problem-solving and the advantages of a troubleshooting mindset. You should have plenty of examples that can be structured as case studies for in-house presentations or possibly for a workshop at your state association. At the senior management level, many decisions involve either financial concerns or personnel issues. While these problems are not normally viewed as behavioral in nature, a deeper dive would suggest that underneath these traditional management concerns are ordinary human behaviors that have gone awry. Taking a behavioral approach to solving a finance problem would by most accounts be considered a *creative* tactic. Issues like inadequate staffing, poor communication, lack of teamwork, and time management at the middle-management level are inherently behavior problems. Applying what you know about behavior analysis and contingency management in a creative way at the top level of a company could be a huge reward for years of seeking creative solutions to individual and team-level challenges.

SUMMARY

This chapter describes a variety of ways that creative problem-solving and troubleshooting can be used in behavior analysis over the span of one's career. As a new BCBA, the focus of problem-solving will likely be on dealing with client behavior problems that cannot be solved using current methods of analysis. We suggest using a series of thought experiments that require you to consider how you might deal with the problem if you had unlimited resources. Or, if you have a successful solution, imagine how you might apply it in different situations such as using the logic of functional analysis with problems like staff turnover or increasing the diversity of your staff members. Troubleshooting involves analyzing each element of a current solution to determine if one or more parts have not been implemented according to plan. This works by asking the question: what can go wrong? For example, the behavior-change plan could be fundamentally sound but if the timing of the delivery of the reinforcers is off, or if the step-size of the task analysis is too large, the plan will likely fail.

FOR FURTHER READING

Creative problem solving. *Wikipedia*. Retrieved January 17, 2021, from https://en.wikipedia.org/wiki/Creative_problem-solving

Creative problem solving: Finding innovative solutions to challenges. *MindTools*. Retrieved January 17, 2021, from www.mindtools.com/pages/article/creative-problem-solving.htm

de Bono, E. (2008). *Creativity workout: 62 exercises to unlock your most creative ideas*. Berkeley, CA: Ulysses Press.

Michalko, M. (2001). *Cracking creativity: The secrets of creative genius*. Berkeley, CA: Ten Speed Press.

Silber, L. (1999). *Career management for the creative person*. New York: Three Rivers Press.

What is creative problem solving? *Creative Education Foundation*. Retrieved January 17, 2021, from www.creativeeducationfoundation.org/what-is-cps/

REFERENCES

Biro, M. M. (2020, July 13). *5 essential soft skills in the workplace*. Retrieved from www.indeed.com/lead/5-soft-skills-in-the-workplace?gclid=EAIaIQobChMIq7WGhMf7-AIV7_bjBx3PtgbVEAAYASAAEgJJf_D_BwE&aceid=

Iwata, B. A., Dorsey, M. F., Slifer, K. J., Bauman, K. E., & Richman, G. S. (1994). Toward a functional analysis of self-injury. *Journal of Applied Behavior Analysis, 27*, 197–209. http://doi.org/10.1901/jaba.1994.27-197

Mager, R. (1975). *Preparing instructional objectives* (2nd ed.). Belmont, CA: Lake Publishing Co.

Mager, R. (1988). *Making instruction work*. Belmont, CA: Lake Publishing Co.

Mager, R., & Pipe, P. (1984). *Analyzing performance problems, or you really oughta wanna* (2nd ed.). Belmont, CA: Lake Publishing Co.

Nalebuff, B., & Ayres, I. (2006). *Why not? How to use everyday ingenuity to solve problems big and small*. Boston: Harvard Business School Press.

Wilder, D. A., Chen, L., Atwell, J., Pritchard, J., & Weinstein, P. (2006). Brief functional analysis and treatment of tantrums associated with transitions in preschool children. *Journal of Applied Behavior Analysis, 39*, 103–107.

22

Insurance and Billing

Michele Silcox-Beal

> ***At least 200 million people now have health insurance coverage for ABA due to our efforts and dedicated advocates across the country. Over the last decade, our advocacy team has focused on improving health insurance coverage for medically necessary treatments such as Applied Behavior Analysis (ABA).***[1]
>
> **—Autism Speaks**

With the increase in health insurance coverage comes a great deal of responsibility for behavior analysts and organizations. Since there are limited courses that specifically train on healthcare insurance and billing while behavior analysts are in college, they can educate themselves independently on key areas of the full revenue cycle management (RCM) process to be successful in their jobs. RCM refers to the process from beginning to end of a health plan. It includes the beneficiary services reimbursed by a health insurance funder.

DOI: 10.4324/9781003265573-27

REVENUE CYCLE MANAGEMENT

- *Payer Contracts and Credentialing*
- *Health Plan Member Benefits and Patient Cost-Shares*
- *Health Plan Service Authorizations*
- *Patient Electronic Health Records*
- *Documentation of Services*
- *Claims submission and reimbursement*
- *Compliance Programs and Preparing for Payer Audits*

FRESH OUT OF GRAD SCHOOL, FIRST JOB AND YOUNG PROFESSIONAL (3–5 YEARS)

Payer Contracts and Credentialing

A behavior analyst partners with payers (the health plan funder) through an organization to complete a credentialing process and become approved to provide services to members (clients/patients) for individual health plans. Once the behavior analyst is board certified, i.e., BCBA, they should apply for an NPI number. The National Provider Identifier (NPI) is a Health Insurance Portability and Accountability Act (HIPAA) Administrative Simplification Standard. The NPI is a unique identification number for covered healthcare providers. This number will stay with an individual provider for the life of their career and be used during credentialing and claims submission. Additionally, with board certification and an NPI number, a behavior analyst should complete the CAQH profile. CAQH is the Council for Affordable Quality Healthcare, Inc., a not-for-profit collaborative alliance of the nation's leading health plans and networks. It is an online data repository of credentialing data. Behavior analysts update demographic, education and training, work history, malpractice history, and other relevant credentialing information for health plans to access during the credentialing process. Consider the CAQH as an online healthcare résumé. It remains with healthcare providers for the duration of their careers and is continuously updated and attested. When a behavior analyst is employed by an organization (practice), the practice information is included in the profile. A behavior analyst can attach more than one practice to their profile. Health plan funders (payers) will also require proof of liability insurance and the organization's Tax ID, and they may have other specific requirements for their plans such as background checks. There are several states that also require licensure. Information regarding state licensure can be found at www.bacb.com/u-s-licensure-of-behavior-analysts/

Recap on what is needed for a behavior analyst to begin billing an insurance company for services:

- *NPI number*
- *CAQH profile*
- *Professional Liability Insurance*
- *Organization Tax ID*
- *State licensure, where applicable*
- *Other requested or required information from individual payers*

Health Plan Member Benefits

A new behavior analyst should familiarize themselves with basic healthcare terminology. A member's (client/patient) benefits for their health plan will include client/patient cost-shares for copays or deductible and co-insurance up to an out-of-pocket maximum. When working with families, having a basic understanding of common healthcare terms will help the behavior analyst navigate concerns from families and partner with the organization's administrative intake team in keeping families informed of their financial responsibility.

The Centers for Medicare and Medicaid Services (CMS) regulates reimbursement for healthcare products and services. CMS resource for some healthcare coverage and terms:

www.cms.gov/cciio/resources/files/downloads/dwnlds/uniform-glossary-final.pdf

As described in the BACB Ethics Code for Behavior Analysts, 3.05 Financial Agreements (see 1.04, 2.07).[2]

> Before beginning services, behavior analysts document agreed-upon compensation and billing practices with their clients, relevant stakeholders, and/or funders. When funding circumstances change, they must be revisited with these parties. Pro bono and bartered services are only provided under a specific service agreement and in compliance with the Code.

Health Plan Service Authorizations

Applied behavior analysis (ABA) services require pre-certification or authorization from a health plan. Behavior analysts should familiarize themselves with Adaptive Behavior Services, aka the ABA Category I CPT® codes used for the authorization of medically necessary services and claims submission for reimbursement from payers. Detailed information can be found at The ABA Coding Coalition website www.abacodes.org. Behavior analysts follow the process for a Behavior Identification Assessment that results in an individualized treatment plan for the patient. CPT® codes are included in the treatment plan to identify the services that need authorization from the health plan to render medically necessary services.

Recap: For a behavior analyst to get pre-certification or authorization from a health plan,

- *Complete Initial and Concurrent service Assessments*
- *Include CPT® codes to match the needs of the individualized treatment plan*
- *Request authorization for ongoing services*
- *Complete Re-Assessment and repeat the authorization process at intervals required by payers (e.g., every six months)*

Patient Electronic Health Records

Behavior analysts have a responsibility to maintain information that is added to the Electronic Health Record (EHR) for patients. An EHR is an electronic version of the patient's medical history across the lifespan of care. www.cms.gov/Medicare/E-Health/EHealthRecords

As described in the BACB Ethics Code for Behavior Analysts, 2.05 Documentation Protection and Retention:

> Behavior analysts are knowledgeable about and comply with all applicable requirements (e.g., BACB rules, laws, regulations, contracts, funder and organization requirements) for storing, transporting, retaining, and destroying physical and electronic documentation related to their professional activities. They destroy physical documentation after making electronic copies or summaries of data (e.g., reports and graphs) only when allowed by applicable requirements. When a behavior analyst leaves an organization, these responsibilities remain with the organization.

Documentation of Services

Behavior analysts are responsible for documenting each client/patient encounter, in the form of a session note, completely, accurately and in a timely manner.

> www.cms.gov/Medicare-Medicaid-Coordination/Fraud-Prevention/Medicaid-Integrity-Program/Education/Documentation

As described in the BACB Ethics Code for Behavior Analysts, 3.11 Documenting Professional Activity (see 1.04, 2.03, 2.05, 2.06, 2.10),

> Throughout the service relationship, behavior analysts create and maintain detailed and high-quality documentation of their professional activities to facilitate provision of services by them or by other professionals, to ensure accountability, and to meet applicable requirements (e.g., laws, regulations, funder and organization policies). Documentation must be created and maintained in a manner that allows for timely communication and transition of services, should the need arise.

As described in the BACB Ethics Code for Behavior Analysts, 2.02 Timeliness:

> Behavior analysts deliver services and carry out necessary service-related administrative responsibilities in a timely manner.

Behavior analysts need to familiarize themselves with the payer policies for any health plans where they will provide services to members (patients). Payer policies generally provide guidance for medical necessity, prior authorization requirements, preadmission guidelines, therapy requirements, and other payer specific information.

Claims Submission and Reimbursement

As described in the BACB Ethics Code for Behavior Analysts, 2.06 Accuracy in Service Billing and Reporting . . .

> Behavior analysts identify their services accurately and include all required information on reports, bills, invoices, requests for reimbursement, and receipts. They do not implement or bill nonbehavioral services under an authorization or contract for behavioral services. If inaccuracies in reporting or billing are discovered, they inform all relevant parties (e.g., organizations, licensure boards, funders), correct the inaccuracy in a timely manner, and document all actions taken in this circumstance and the eventual outcomes.

By following the steps covered in this section and adhering to the BACB Ethics Code and payer requirements, behavior analysts will be prepared to submit information to a health plan in the form of a medical claim for reimbursement of rendered services.

Compliance Programs and Preparing for Payer Audits

In 1993, the Attorney General made tackling healthcare fraud one of the Department's top priorities. The Department continues to upgrade its efforts in combatting the full array of fraud perpetrated by healthcare providers. CMS provides a variety of resources on how to detect, prevent and report fraud, waste, and abuse.

> www.cms.gov/Outreach-and-Education/Medicare-Learning-Network-MLN/MLNProducts/Downloads/Fraud-Abuse-MLN4649244.pdf

The False Claims Act (FCA) in the healthcare sector imposes liability on any person who submits a claim to the federal government that he or she knows (or should know) is false.

www.justice.gov/civil/false-claims-act

The creation of compliance program guidance remains a major effort by the Office of Inspector General (OIG) in its effort to engage the healthcare community in combating fraud and abuse.

In formulating compliance guidance, the OIG has worked closely with the Health Care Financing Administration (HCFA), the Department of Justice (DOJ) and various sectors of the healthcare industry to provide clear guidance to those segments of the industry that are interested in reducing fraud and abuse within their organizations.

https://oig.hhs.gov/documents/compliance-guidance/801/physician.pdf

Behavior analysts should participate in and support a culture of compliance. Health plans will periodically audit billing and documentation; therefore, compliance cannot be an afterthought. Having a compliance program, ongoing training, and internal audits will help keep behavior analysts and organizations out of harm's way of fraudulent activity.

MID-CAREER (6–10 YEARS) AND SENIOR BEHAVIOR ANALYST

At this career level, a behavior analyst may have already been assigned supervisor responsibilities or promoted to clinical leadership. This may be the time when a seasoned behavior analyst makes the decision regarding business ownership, expanding the scope of accountability.

This can be the career level where the behavior analyst develops relationships with provider representatives for the health plan funders where contracts exist. Having these relationships can be advantageous for negotiating rates, sharing the value of your organization's services for the members of the health plan. It can also be helpful when there is a pattern of erroneous claims denials or systemic issues with claims processing in the health plan system. Provider representatives can advocate on behalf of the payer and assist in navigating through issues.

With oversight or ownership responsibilities, behavior analysts must consider the seriousness of contractual responsibilities and their own personal or business liability. It is imperative that leaders and owners put processes in place to ensure that services are documented adequately, and claims are submitted ethically and in compliance with healthcare standards, contractual obligations, and payer requirements. Failure to pass a payer audit can result in recoupments, possible fines, and loss of contracts.

Section G of the False Claims Act (FCA) is known as the Reverse False Claims section. It provides liability where a person acts improperly to avoid paying money owed to the government for overpayments. An overpayment can also be for a claim paid where the services were billed incorrectly due to lack of appropriate documentation, incorrect coding, or not following the CPT® code guidelines.

An effective and successful compliance plan *and* maintaining a culture of compliance is the responsibility of leadership. A compliance plan should outline each of the seven elements and include directions, standards, and policies for how each element is handled. If an area of non-compliance is found, detailed records of the incident or misconduct should be documented with the date, name of the person that reported the issue, the person who initialed action on the issue, and any corrective or follow-up action that was taken.

Seasoned behavior analysts should be able to perform the following for the organization's compliance plan:

- Identify how each role/function can contribute to mitigating risk
- Document, disseminate, train, and test all processes, policies, and procedures
- Include feedback and participation from team members

- Set up an Audit schedule and complete audits
- Adjust where necessary, educate and provide continuous feedback
- Revisit and update processes, policies, and procedures on a regular cycle

Behavior analysts in clinical leadership or as owners should take care to educate themselves fully on the areas covered in this chapter to ensure they are training and providing appropriate guidance to their supervisees or employees. At this level of your career, you have the opportunity to contribute to providing accurate information and training to other behavior analysts in the field and demonstrating ethical and compliant billing practices to health plan funders.

SUMMARY

This chapter outlined key aspects of working with health insurance companies. Behavior analysts need to be able to navigate health insurance services and billing at all four stages of their careers from graduate students to senior behavior analysts. Working with health plan funders (payers) can be complicated and overwhelming. Behavior analysts must be well informed about contracts, credentialing, payer relationships, patient health plan benefits, service authorizations, full-cycle claims reimbursement, and compliance. They can actively support a culture of compliance within an organization that has industry billing knowledge, health plan requirements, and responsibilities for working with payers in the medical model. As a behavior analyst grows in experience and chooses to open a private practice or is promoted to clinical leadership, the burden of responsibility increases for other providers within the organization. Having a solid understanding of the elements of this chapter will lay the foundation for increased responsibilities in a behavior analyst's career. Given that there is a wide variety in the field for the timeline of when a behavior analyst may take on additional responsibility, it is recommended that each section be studied, reviewed, and applied based on individual circumstances.

NOTES

1 www.autismspeaks.org/health-insurance-coverge-autism
2 Behavior Analyst Certification Board. (2020). *Ethics code for behavior analysts.* Retrieved from https://bacb.com/wp-content/ethics-code-for-behavior-analysts/

FOR FURTHER READING

Silcox, M., & Schmitz, S. (2019). *Revenue cycle management—ABA therapy.* Hayes, VA: Cape Cod Collaboration.

23
Critical Thinking

We cannot solve our problems with the same thinking we used when we created them.
—Albert Einstein

FRESH OUT OF GRAD SCHOOL, FIRST JOB

> Extraordinary claims require extraordinary proof . . .

On your first job as a behavior analyst, as you assemble your team of RBTs and trainees, determine your scope of competence and that of your therapists and technicians, and establish yourself as a professional, you will no doubt be serving as a role model for critical thinking. You will also be an instructor in the fine art of distinguishing myths and fads from evidence-based procedures. Over time you may develop a reputation as someone who sticks to the evidence for each client and determines if a recommended treatment works for them. Critical thinking becomes a way of life, and for the successful behavior analyst, it is automatic.

From the time you take your first job until you become an experienced behavior analyst, you may discover that your basic scientific-method training clashes with that of colleagues who may have been trained less rigorously. The scientific method is founded

DOI: 10.4324/9781003265573-28

in using critical thinking about how the world works. Behavior analysts *are* critical thinkers, skeptics even. We are not pessimists or optimists. Rather we often adhere so close to the line "Where's the data?" that many people in human services sometimes find us to be insensitive or difficult to work with. We always question everything including the methodology and findings in published research (see Bailey & Burch, 2018, pp. 193–195). We also question dramatic personal anecdotes. Because we won't accept a touching story of a new miraculous breakthrough cure for a behavior problem, it might appear that we are basically cynics who don't believe in anything but science. Our unofficial motto, "Extraordinary claims require extraordinary proof"[1] is a good way to express our general approach.

We *do* require everyone who wants to talk about behavior to have data, and not just any data but data acquired through repeated measures, demonstrating IOA (inter-observer agreement), and, of course, social validity. And don't forget, there must be a clear demonstration of experimental control and the data must show a socially significant effect. Behavior analysts are not usually impressed with randomized statistical tests when they are used to draw conclusions about behavior. By this standard, 98% of the evidence about human behavior in the world falls short of our requirements. No other treatment approach comes close to this rigor, and it can make colleagues in related professions, and quite a few consumers, squirm. We are not interested in correlational findings (even if they are statistically significant) that show that boys are better at math than girls or that people who sleep on their backs are repressed (or is it depressed?). We *are* interested in knowing the causal variables surrounding individual human behavior, and we understand that some are proximal (close in), and others are distal (somewhat removed, such as something that happened two months ago). Because we can't control the distal variables, we emphasize the proximal and insist that to *really* understand behavior, we must intervene and treat it systematically. We believe in a treatment only when enough replications have been performed.

Even then, we understand that these findings, perhaps published by reputable applied scientists in our flagship journal, may not directly apply to our current client. In these cases, we insist on taking a baseline for each client behavior, testing the intervention, and determining for ourselves if it works in *this* setting for *this* individual. As it turns out, we are intermittently reinforced for all this critical thinking, as it frequently happens that treatments that sound too good to be true are not (true). And it happens every day that we try a published procedure with a client and discover, for some reason, it doesn't work. We have mixed emotions over this. Although we wished that the treatment had worked and were disappointed that it didn't, we were certainly glad our baseline and subsequent data collection objectively evaluated the treatment.

Casual Thinking Versus Critical Thinking

Most thinking that we engage in daily is not *critical* thinking at all but simple *casual* thinking: "It's time for an oil change; I go right past a Jiffy Lube® on my way home from work, so I guess I'll stop and get done today." Critical thinking would involve asking whether frequent lubrication is required as part of maintenance (the intervals depend on the type of car, be sure to consult the manual that came with it) and what type of oil has been demonstrated to be the most effective (Barrera, 2021).

> The real problem occurs when you allow yourself to be lulled into mushy, casual thinking when valuable time, money, and opportunity costs are at stake and your clients are involved.

Other routine, casual (non-critical) thinking may involve taking advice from a friend, "You must try this Fair-Trade Organic Sumatran Reserve coffee. It has the most amazing flavor and aroma and is grown in soil that has never been treated with pesticides, so you won't get cancer from it." It takes some effort to do critical thinking on matters such as this and depending on whether you share your critical thinking with others, you might not be too popular. People like to influence one another, and if you analyze your friend's recommendations and critique their advice, there is a good chance they will replace you with another friend. In most cases on a day-by-day basis, *casual* thinking is perfectly fine. You can usually get along without any serious damage to your friendships, although you might buy an occasional over-hyped, overpriced bag of coffee that tastes exactly like Folgers®. The real problem occurs when you allow yourself to be lulled into mushy, casual thinking when valuable time, money, and opportunity costs are at stake and your clients are involved.

Critical Thinking in Action

Our version of critical thinking, having evolved directly from our single-case experimental method and honed over five decades in applied settings and university laboratories, has left us with a legacy of skepticism about non-behavioral theories and treatments. We encounter these theories about behavior daily in our role as professionals, and new, wilder theories are introduced nearly every day. From chiropractic manipulations to improve the nervous system, to chelation administrations to remove heavy metals from the body to gluten- and casein-free diets that allege to reduce peptide levels and improve behavior and cognitive functioning, new untested beliefs abound (Foxx, 2010). Failure to use critical thinking in these instances could result in harm to a client and a major hit on the client's bank account, not to mention a substantial amount of time wasted that could have been put toward evidence-based treatments. Many families desperate for any shred of hope for a *cure* for autism seem disinclined to engage in critical thinking about treatment effectiveness, but Freeman

We encounter theories about behavior daily in our role as professionals, and new theories are being announced nearly every day.

(2007) has shown a path forward in her book *The Complete Guide to Autism Treatments*.

We can look at one very popular treatment, sensory integration (SI), as a way of showing what would be involved in casually vs. critically thinking about an untested theory. SI, a widely popular theory, was introduced in 1972 (Ayres, 1972). The claim is that the integration of stimuli from the body and the environment requires a "balance between excitatory and inhibitory neurological systems" (Bundy & Murray, 2002). Sensory integrative therapy (SIT) includes engaging in activities to stimulate the vestibular system, such as being pushed in a swing or rolled on a mat, or riding on scooter boards (Smith, Mruzek, & Mozingo, 2005, pp. 331–332). Other activities such as squeezing the client between gym pads to provide "deep pressure" or brushing them with a soft brush are postulated to therapeutically stimulate the proprioceptive or tactile systems of the individual. As far-fetched as this therapy sounds, supporters of SIT claim that these treatments enhance the individual's ability to focus on materials, reduce their maladaptive behavior, and lead to improvements in nervous system functioning (Smith et al., 2005, p. 332), and yet direct, observable, measurable data is lacking.

Casual thinking might go like this: "The theory has been around a long time, there is some research on it, and occupational therapists recommend it, why not try it?"

Critical thinking (Paul & Elder, 2012) requires people to separate *information* (data) from their *assumptions* about the information. We need to be able to see a straight line from *data* to *inferences* (conclusions), recognizing our assumptions and reducing them to a minimum. Finally, we must understand that the inferences we make have *implications* (consequences), in this case the implications for the client (see Figure 23.1). To accept this theory without critically investigating the published research and without evaluating it for our individual clients is a clear example of uncritical thinking that can lead to wasted time, squandered resources, and worst of all, false hope.

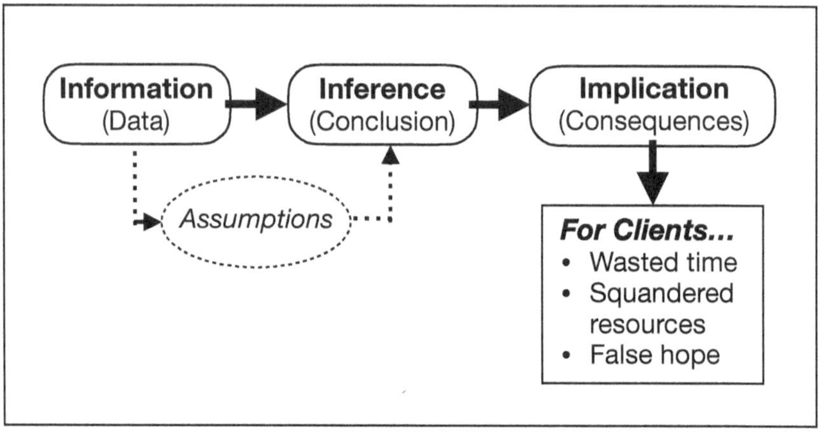

Figure 23.1 This flowchart shows critical thinking steps, including the role that assumptions can play in the critical thinking process and the consequences for clients.

Adapted with permission from Paul, R. W., & Elder, L. (2012). *Critical thinking: Tools for taking charge of your learning and your life*. Boston, MA: Pearson Education, Inc.

Therapists who employ SIT are applying the method in the absence of any experimental data that proves it is effective; they are simply assuming the theory is correct. Unfortunately, this leads to their spending hours and hours engaged in wasteful and repetitious brushing, swinging, and squeezing of their clients to no avail. Consumers of these services are clearly not engaging in critical thinking—if they were, they would be asking the occupational therapist, "Is that true? Can you give me more details on that? Does this really make sense?" Consumers cannot be expected to be knowledgeable about research methodology or theories involving the nervous system. They are at the mercy of these professionals to properly, honestly, characterize the treatment approach. There is a certain amount of sophistry going on here as well; supporters of SIT should be aware that their research is weak and inconclusive.[2] In a detailed analysis of this body of work, Smith et al. (2005, p. 345) concluded, "Studies indicate that SIT is ineffective and that its theoretical underpinnings and assessment practices are unvalidated."

One early behavioral study done with sensory integration (SI) as an independent variable (Mason & Iwata, 1990) was carried out with the specific purpose of testing SI theory. Results showed that none of the three participants improved with SI treatment. The data for one participant are shown in Figure 23.2 for illustrative purposes.[3] Kathy clearly showed a paradoxical effect; that is, she showed increased self-injurious behaviors when the SI procedures were put in place, which certainly was not an expected outcome but one that indicates that such essentially untested, but great-sounding, methods can in fact do some harm. More recently SI theory was tested in treating children with feeding disorders and found to be far less effective than a behavior analytic approach (Addison et al., 2013; Peterson, Piazza, & Volkert, 2016).

Lives were ruined by FC when innocent people spent months in jail until a proper hearing and testimony from experts could be provided.

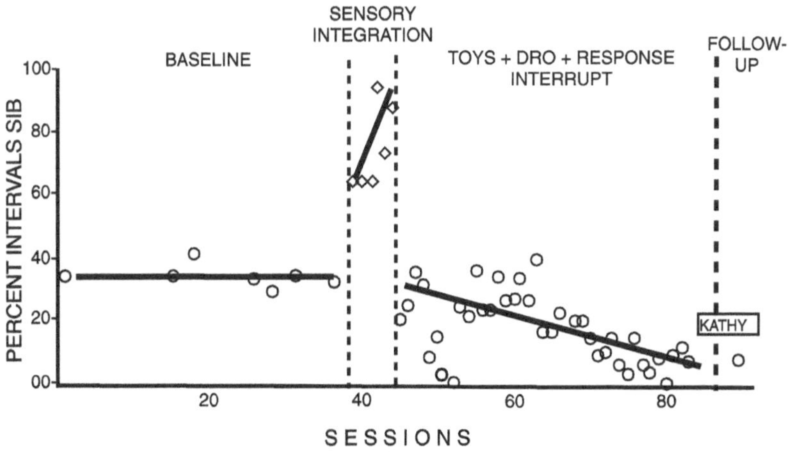

Figure 23.2 Data for one participant from the Mason and Iwata (1990) study.

Data are redrawn to illustrate the effects of the sensory integration procedures more clearly. From Mason, S. A., & Iwata, B. A. (1990). Artifactual effects of sensory-integrative therapy on self-injurious behavior. *Journal of Applied Behavior Analysis*, *23*, 361–370.

Facilitated Communication: The Poster Child for Failed Critical Thinking

Perhaps the greatest debacle tied to a failure of critical thinking involved Facilitated Communication (FC), a fad treatment if ever there was one. FC began in Australia as a treatment for individuals with cerebral palsy and then migrated to the United States in the early 1990s as a method for assisting communication for people with autism (Jacobson, Foxx, & Mulick, 2005; Foxx & Mulick, 2016). The assumption is that individuals with autism have "undisclosed literacy" and that a facilitator can assist them in bringing out their latent literary talents by helping them type on a keyboard to express themselves. It wouldn't take much critical thinking to bring this observation (and assumption) to its knees, so it is surprising that FC caught on and spread like wildfire in the late 1990s. In an experimental analysis of FC published in the *Journal of Applied Behavior Analysis* (Montee, Miltenberger, & Wittrock, 1995) the researchers clearly showed that "the facilitators controlled the typing" (p. 197).

> For you as a behavior analyst, critical thinking tools are essential every time you go to work.

So desperate and trusting were the consumers (i.e., counselors, school administrators, family members) that facilitators were hired at school system expense to sit with severely and profoundly mentally handicapped individuals and help them write poetry, express lifestyle preferences, and, in several cases, allege crimes against relatives. Even the judicial system failed in its critical thinking skills to see the obvious: It was the facilitators who were writing the short stories and doing the math problems. One dead giveaway was that the individuals who were being facilitated did not appear in the least to be interested in the task and often were observed to be looking in the opposite direction of the keyboard (Foxx, 1994). Instead of asking critical questions about the procedures, advocates for FC *assumed* that they were capable of self-advocacy, thus totally distorting the information right in front of them. The consequences (see Figure 23.1) have been devastating for families that were ripped apart by fallacious allegations. Lives were ruined by FC when innocent people spent months in jail until a proper hearing and testimony from experts could be provided (Maurice, Green, & Luce, 1996).

Critical Thinking Goes to Work

For you as a behavior analyst, critical thinking tools are essential every time you go to work. Teachers, parents, and administrators will describe some horrendous situation that requires your immediate attention and will confront you at least weekly: "Drop everything and take care of this!" It is usually a third-hand story about some individual who is in desperate need of "behavior modification." Your job is to remain calm, review the evidence, determine what assumptions have been made and by whom, and do your level best to arrive at a reasoned conclusion. People on the front lines have been reinforced for exaggerating their claims and embellishing their stories. Anything less will get a shrug and a smile and little else. Most people do not have data to give you to quantify the problem, and colorful anecdotes full of dramatic details designed to spur you to action are the modus operandi. You must be especially careful not to believe the first story you hear but rather to reserve your judgment until you've heard from all parties. Then, in full critical thinking mode, try to sort out what happened and arrive at a conclusion. If you want to remain true to your behavior analysis tradition, you will need to establish some sort of actual baseline before you draw any conclusions. Establishing this baseline is key to critical thinking in applied behavior analysis and will no doubt cause consternation among those who want immediate action.

The second challenge to your critical thinking will come when you devise an intervention based on your functional analysis and implement a treatment. Because it is *your* treatment plan, you will be inclined to like it and believe it will work. You will need to put on your critical thinking hat here and evaluate your plan objectively, setting aside your assumption that "Of course, it will work, I designed it. Why wouldn't it work?" The correction against going easy on yourself is to submit your program and data to a peer-review committee and receive feedback on a regular basis.

Critical thinking also comes into play every time you open a journal to research the current best practices in behavior analysis. Although we usually think of "published in a peer-reviewed journal" as the standard for evidence-based practice, experience has shown that a significant number of such studies fall short, way short. Applying critical thinking to these studies reveals that many simply don't meet our standards. Baselines are too short or too variable, the dependent variable is not well defined, the IOA is below 80%, conditions are not replicated, the size of effect is too small to be socially significant, and more. Research conducted in the first author's Behavior Analysis Research Lab (Normand & Bailey, 2006) showed that participants, all Board Certified Behavior Analysts®, made accurate decisions for only 72% of the graphs they reviewed. Even the addition of celeration lines did not improve overall accuracy. If BCBAs (presumably well trained at the master's level) are unable to properly analyze published studies and determine which are suitable as a basis for building an effective treatment plan, we have a critical thinking problem in our profession.

YOUNG PROFESSIONAL (3–5 YEARS)

As a more mature young professional who has trained countless therapists in critical thinking methods, you should be ready for the next phase—spreading the word throughout your organization. You may have already been tapped to supervise new BCBAs who may not have been exposed to critical thinking in the practice of behavior analysis. With several years of experience behind you, now you should be able to recount examples where you had to gently confront a family that firmly believed in FC or its offspring the RPM (Rapid Prompting Method), which has also been disproven (Lang, Tostanoski, Travers, & Todd, 2014), and they wanted you to include it as part of the treatment package for their child. Using all your persuasion skills (see Chapter 2 in this book on interpersonal skills) hopefully, you were able to convince them that this was little more than a bogus fad treatment and that their time would be better spent learning how to apply basic behavior shaping techniques (see Chapter 12 on shaping). Instituting a monthly journal reading group is another way to spread the word about critical thinking. You can assign articles that purport to offer a behavior change method that on closer scrutiny does not meet our high standards for evidence (see Bailey & Burch, 2018, pp. 199–201, Evaluating Behavioral Research).

MID-CAREER (6–10 YEARS)

At mid-career, you may well have moved up to a middle management position in your organization. This will give you a broader scope of influence. For example, those monthly journal reading group meetings could be made a required part of in-house training for all therapists, techs, BCaBAs, and BCBAs. A requirement that all behavior plans employed by your organization include references to *JABA* quality research studies as part of the justification for their inclusion might also be instituted.

SENIOR BEHAVIOR ANALYST

With years of experience as a behavior analyst and a champion for critical thinking, you may now be able to help your organization or company to think more broadly about policies and procedures that may be out of date or nonfunctional. After all, critical thinking does not just apply to behavior analysis but also to purchasing, marketing, recruiting, finance, company growth, communication, and strategic planning. For example, a critical look at marketing may show that too much revenue is going to this department with meager results, or your company's recruitment strategy may not have kept up with the times as demographics show the pool of potential RBTs has changed since the company was founded.

SUMMARY

This chapter presents an argument for the rigorous application of critical thinking in the field of behavior analysis. As we are besieged with fads, crazy controversial theories, and unvalidated treatments, the need for critical thinking is more important than ever. When presented with a new treatment proposal, behavior analysts employ critical thinking by asking "Where's the data?" Taking advice without question is an example of casual thinking and is common in daily life where the stakes are not high. Sensory integration is one commonly used treatment that does not have the support of the behavioral community since the research does not meet our rigorous standards. Facilitated Communication is another "treatment" that has been shown to be phony, as the research has shown the key-pad responses actually represent the behavior of the facilitator rather than the client. We have rigorous methodological standards for ABA research because it has produced the highest level of evidence-based treatment.

NOTES

1 https://en.wikipedia.org/wiki/Marcello_Truzzi
2 *Sophistry* is a specious argument used for deceiving someone.
3 The data have been redrawn to isolate the effects for one client, Kathy. In the original figure, hers is the middle graph of three in a multiple baseline design.

FOR FURTHER READING

Zechmeister, E. B., & Johnson, J. E. (1992). *Critical thinking: A functional approach*. Pacific Grove, CA: Brooks/Cole.

REFERENCES

Addison, L. R., Piazza, C. C., Patel, M. R., Bachmeyer, M. H., Rivas, K. M., Milnes, S. S., & Oddo, J. (2013). A comparison of sensory integrative and behavioral therapies as treatment for pediatric feeding disorders. *Journal of Applied Behavior Analysis*, *45*(3).

Ayres, A. J. (1972). *Sensory integration and learning disorders.* Los Angeles: Western Psychological Services.
Bailey, J. S., & Burch, M. R. (2018). *Research methods in applied behavior analysis* (2nd ed.). New York: Routledge, Inc.
Barrera, A. (2021). *Best motor oils for 2022.* Retrieved from www.forbes.com/wheels/accessories/best-motor-oils/
Bundy, A. C., & Murray, E. A. (2002). Assessing sensory integrative dysfunction. In A. C. Bundy, S. J. Lane, & A. Murray (Eds.), *Sensory integration: Theory and practice* (2nd ed., pp. 3–34). Philadelphia: Davis.
Foxx, R. M. (1994, Fall). Facilitated communication in Pennsylvania: Scientifically invalid but politically correct. *Dimensions*, 1–9.
Foxx, R. M. (2010). The complete guide to autism treatments: A parent's handbook. *Behavior Analysis in Practice.* Spring, *33*(1), 133–138.
Foxx, R. M., & Mulick, J. A. (Eds.). (2016). *Controversial therapies for developmental disabilities: Fad, fashion, and science in professional practice* (2nd ed.). New York: Routledge, Inc.
Freeman, S. K. (2007). *The complete guide to autism treatments: A parent's handbook: Make sure your child gets what works*! Lynden, WA: SKF Books.
Jacobson, J. W., Foxx, R. M., & Mulick, J. A. (Eds.). (2005). *Controversial therapies for developmental disabilities.* Mahwah, NJ: Lawrence Erlbaum Associates Publishers.
Lang, R., Tostanoski, A. H., Travers, J., & Todd, J. (2014). The only study investigating the rapid prompting method has serious methodological flaws but data suggest the most likely outcome is prompt dependency. *Evidence-Based Communication Assessment and Intervention*, *8*(1), 40–48. http://doi.org/10.1080/17489539.2014.955260
Mason, S. A., & Iwata, B. A. (1990). Artifactual effects of sensory-integrative therapy on self-injurious behavior. *Journal of Applied Behavior Analysis, 23*, 361–370.
Maurice, C., Green, G., & Luce, S. C. (Eds.). (1996). *Behavioral intervention for young children with autism: A manual for parents and professionals.* Austin, TX: PRO-ED.
Montee, B. B., Miltenberger, R. G., & Wittrock, D. (1995). An experimental analysis of facilitated communication. *Journal of Applied Behavior Analysis, 28*(2), 189–200.
Normand, M. T., & Bailey, J. S. (2006). The effects of celeration lines on accurate data analysis. *Behavior Modification, 30*, 295–314.
Paul, R. W., & Elder, L. (2012). *Critical thinking: Tools for taking charge of your learning and your life.* Boston, MA: Pearson Education, Inc.

Peterson, K. M., Piazza, C. C., & Volkert, V. M. (2016). A comparison of a modified sequential oral sensory approach to an applied behavior-analytic approach in the treatment of food selectivity in children with autism spectrum disorder. *Journal of Applied Behavior Analysis*, *49*(3).

Smith, T., Mruzek, D. W., & Mozingo, D. (2005). Sensory integrative therapy. In J. W. Jacobson, R. M. Foxx, & J. A. Mulick (Eds.), *Controversial therapies for developmental disabilities*. Mahwah, NJ: Lawrence Erlbaum Associates.

24
Design Thinking

Think Different!

—Steve Jobs

FRESH OUT OF GRAD SCHOOL, FIRST JOB

Introduction to Design Thinking

When you were in graduate school, odds are that you never heard of *Design Thinking* because it is a field totally apart from behavior analysis. Likewise, professionals who use this methodology have probably never heard of ABA. We firmly believe that this unique method of understanding human performance processes and how it can be used to improve the delivery of services is totally relevant to our field. Design thinking has been around since 1990 and has been used to improve a wide variety of products and services from the Oral B toothbrush to Netflix ("5 examples of design thinking in business," n.d.) and Airbnb to IBM and Bank of America ("8 great design thinking examples," n.d.). *Design thinking* is billed as *human-centric* in that the focus from the very initial steps is on the consumer and how they interact with the product or service. The data is accumulated through surveys, questionnaires, and direct observation. Rather than make assumptions about what the consumer knows or exactly how they would use the product or service, designers choose to learn directly from the consumer.

DOI: 10.4324/9781003265573-29

In the case of behavior analysis, we have several types of *consumers* we train on behavioral-clinical skills including the client, their caregivers, and stakeholders. We also have teachers, aides, administrators, and other school employees who may need to be trained to use behavioral principles and procedures. The list goes on to include non-behavioral colleagues such as speech therapists or counselors who may be involved in using behavior techniques in their practice. Behavior analysts working in business and industry (OBM/PM) are routinely training mid-level managers, line supervisors, and executives on behavioral methods geared toward non-clinical applications that are designed to improve safety, reduce waste, and improve efficiency and productivity.

In the clinical setting, our current methodology is to conduct an assessment and an interview with the stakeholders (which hopefully drives a search for evidence-based methods of treatment), prepare a technically and terminologically correct written treatment plan, gain approval from caregivers or other associates, and somehow put the plan in place. We have some rudimentary ideas of how to train RBTs on these plans, but the idea of looking at such a complex set of instructions and contingencies from their perspective would be considered unusual at best. The same goes for training parents. While there are some exceptions, parent training usually ranges from handing parents a 20-page plan full of jargon, to having them listen to a talk about reinforcement during an hour-long lecture in a room with a dozen other parents.

> Designers use the term *empathy* to describe this process because they feel it helps them put aside their personal assumptions and focus on the part of the customer's life that they want to improve.

We believe that as a new BCBA, there are many tips and strategies you could learn from this field (Brown, 2009). These strategies could have a great impact on the way in which you train the RBTs and caregivers who are expected to implement the behavior plans

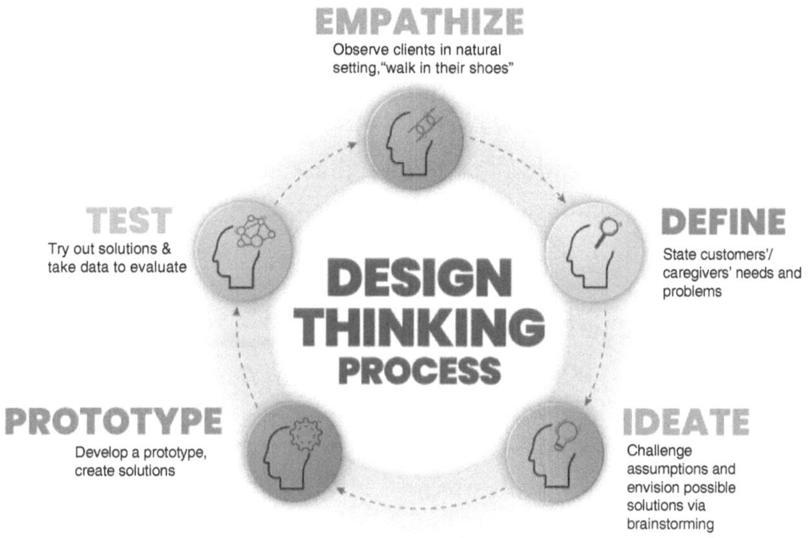

Figure 24.1 This graphic shows the five-step process of Design Thinking.

that you have so carefully crafted. They essentially become your most immediate consumers. Depending on which books you read, there are either five or six (or more) steps (Lewrick, Link, & Leifer, 2018; Dam, 2022) in design thinking. We will outline these in basic terms and indicate how we think they would fit with our behavior analysis way of thinking and methodology.

Step 1. Empathize (Discover Your Consumer's Needs)

At this initial stage of the process, the goal is to learn as much as possible about your consumer/client, their daily routine, their habits, and their priorities. How do they discipline, and what are their expectations for their children's mealtime, play, homework, and especially family time together? Under a typical ABA scenario, the behavior analyst would gather this information in an interview conducted in the office. Recently Helvey and Van Camp (2022) went a little further and made "naturalistic observations" of the caregiver/participant interactions in a padded room at the university clinic. But design thinking professionals want to see for themselves what the home or community environment looks like and what the normal, routine interactions are. Designers use the term *empathy* to describe this process because they feel it helps them put aside their personal assumptions and focus on the part of the customer's life that they want to improve—a perfect match for our goals as contemporary behavior analysts. If the referral was for food refusal, for example, designers would specifically want to observe several mealtimes in the home. If the referral was for non-compliance or aggression, they would find out when this was most likely to occur and make their observations at those times. If designers were consulting with a behavior analyst they would say, "Design your program so that it matches the family's daily routine as much as possible." This brings us to Step 2.

In Step 2, the focus will be on the caregiver's *needs* rather than characteristics of the behavior plan. Designers call this *need-finding*. They will ask, "What does the consumer/caregiver want to achieve?"

Step 2. Define Your Consumer's Needs and Problems

For this step, the goal is to use the substantial information gained in Step 1. This yields a thorough understanding of the problem referral so that you can state with confidence the client's needs for a solution. In behavior analysis, this is usually done by the lone BCBA using the initial interview data plus the assessment results. In design thinking, this would be done by a team that is reviewing all of their notes taken in Step 1.

In Step 2, the focus will be on the caregiver's *needs* rather than the characteristics of the behavior plan. Designers call this *need-finding*. They will ask, "What does the consumer/caregiver want to achieve?"

Additional questions would be, "What will motivate them to use our ideas?" "Is there anything that will prevent them from adopting our behavior plan?" A parent may say, "I want Amory to sit quietly at mealtime, eat politely using proper utensils, and converse with the rest of the family." The detailed, direct observations from Step 1 revealed that Amory did none of this. He would not sit still, ate with his fingers, and after only a few bites left the table to run around the living room. The parents probably have no idea that some of the problem involves the food that is served and their constant aversive sounding prompting, e.g., "Sit down Amory, I told you to sit down, did you hear me? And quit using your fingers, that's ugly, do you want people to think you are an animal . . ." It is obvious that a standard behavior plan that simply *instructs* the caregivers to give effective instructions and implement escape avoidance will likely fail. In the next step, designers will start to generate ideas for parent training; this will include brainstorming sessions and may include, in Amory's case, his family, the caregivers, and possibly other stakeholders (e.g., grandparents, the babysitter, siblings).

This process called *ideation* may involve simple brainstorming, i.e., coming up with as many ideas as possible, with no criticism, and only a large volume of thoughts, inklings, perceptions, and viewpoints.

Step 3. Create Ideas: Challenge Assumptions

In this step, design thinkers are ready to begin the process of generating ideas. They know what the consumers want from Step 1, and they have accumulated numerous observations from Step 2, so they are now ready to help create a *user-centric* statement of the problem. This process called *ideation* may involve simple brainstorming, i.e., coming up with as many ideas as possible, with no criticism, and only a large volume of thoughts, inklings, perceptions, and viewpoints. The leader of the team, most likely the behavior analyst, would conduct two or three brainstorming sessions during which the group puts their ideas on the table for consideration. From a behavior analytic perspective, some of those ideas might look like this: Change the dinnertime arrangement; have Amory eat with just one parent at a separate time from the rest of the family; change the food that is served to things that he enjoys; train that one parent to prompt and reinforce utensil use; have him help prepare the food, etc. For the parents, the team may consider training the parents using a role-play method after watching a video or after watching a therapist have dinner with Amory. Other ideas that the behavior analyst is likely to consider are Amory will probably need some training away from the table, start with food he enjoys, and provide intensive practice with a trained therapist on using a spoon and fork. The parents may need similar separate training on how to give simple instructions along with effective, descriptive reinforcers. From a design thinking perspective, this is the general direction this parent training should take which is quite different from the standard approach.[1]

> *Users* interact with these scenarios, while the designers observe and ask the users for their immediate reactions, summary evaluation, and possible input for changes.

Step 4. Develop Prototype Solutions

Designers often work for companies that are looking to improve the performance of certain apps, kitchen tools, and interactive devices such as the instrument clusters in the new electric vehicles. In this step, designers will take the best ideas generated in Step 3 and develop prototypes which are mock-ups made of simple materials that can be used to test the solutions in a realistic way. For *experiences*, designers will develop narratives, storyboards, or video clips. *Users* interact with these scenarios, while the designers observe and ask the users for their immediate reactions, summary evaluation, and possible input for changes. The behavior analysts-as-designers need to be open to this feedback and prepared to start over if the reaction to their prototype is negative. If the designers are working with customer services, they may use role-play situations to see how users respond. This latter example comes fairly close to what we might do in behavior analysis.

> Questions that need to be answered in this step include: What did the users like about the product or service? What questions did they have? Are there any criticisms of the product or service? Were any new ideas generated out of the test?

The *prototype* step might consist of users responding to a therapist reading a dinner-time scenario, listening to pre-recorded audio of a family's interaction over a meal, viewing video clips of different ways that people handle dinner-time behavior problems, parents receiving BST training, or therapists teaching basic skills. Caregivers might also view a series of real-time role-plays with therapists-as-parents (called *bodystorming*, Lewrick et al., 2018). The therapists interact as a stand-in for Amory and his behavior problems to gain the parent's reactions and feedback. The concept of social validity (Wolf, 1978) stresses the importance of consumer evaluation of goals, procedures, and outcomes in the development of applied behavioral research and it seems totally appropriate as a method to apply at this step of design thinking for behavior analysts.

Out of this prototyping should come the best solution that is likely to make a difference. In behavioral research, we call this *pilot testing*, and it is a common procedure in the development of appropriate, accurate measurement systems, the creation of effective independent variables, and of course the establishment of the important dependent variable (Bailey & Burch, 2018).

Step 5. Test Your Solutions With Your Consumers
For this step, design thinkers will seek out potential customers for their product or service, and if feasible, they will identify the actual context of where the service will be used. The design thinkers will interview users, and just like behavior analysts, they will observe and take data. The data taken by design thinkers is more likely to be descriptive rather than quantitative as in ABA. For example, it might include videotaping the users in action. Even at this stage of design thinking, there is an iterative process, new ideas may come out of the test, or the users may make suggestions that had not been brought up in the prototype phase. Questions that need to be answered in this step include: What did the users like about the product or service? What questions did they have? Are there any criticisms of the product or service? Were any new ideas generated out of the test (Lewrick et al., 2018, p. 123)? This tactic, if applied to ABA, could greatly improve the delivery of behavior programs that are not only effective but appreciated and highly rated by users. This might be called *Social Validity 2.0.*

Designers like to use what they call *A/B Testing* of their prototypes (Lewrick et al., 2018, p. 124); that is, they compare two versions side-by-side and have the consumers judge which they prefer. Our first experience with this approach came early in the field (Iwata & Bailey, 1974) with a study on reward versus cost token systems. In this study, the students preferred reward, but the teacher preferred response cost. For reference, this type of comparison is often carried out with multiple schedules of reinforcement in both lab and applied settings (Pizarro, Vollmer, & Morris, 2021; Nava, Vargo, & Babino, 2016). The work with functional analysis also incorporates this methodology. For example, an isolated FA includes comparisons of several variables using a multi-element design. Recently, this method has been compared with synthesized contingency analysis (SCA) (Helvey & Van Camp, 2022) in an A/B comparison to determine which was better at predicting controlling variables.

We have a need in ABA to do a great deal more in the way of getting user input on some of our procedures and design thinking can provide some creative ways of doing this. We need to reverse our thinking about program development from a *Top Down* approach in which the BCBA decides, to using a *Bottom Up* approach where the consumer has significant input. We have literature on the effects of choice on behavior (Fisher & Mazur, 1997; Hanratty & Hanley, 2021; Brandt, Dozier, Juanico, Laudont, & Mick, 2015). This unique approach involving choice can be expanded beyond the user choosing one of two researcher-developed interventions to the user being involved from the early stages with input into the way new treatment strategies are developed and instituted.

So, what can you do on your first job to promote *design thinking* in your work as a newly minted BCBA? Start by doing some reading on the topic. As you are assigned clinical cases, you might start to think of ways of better understanding the daily routine of your consumers (parents, caregivers, stakeholders) and the contingencies they experience each day. For consumers to get on board with a behavioral approach, they will need to incorporate your ideas for behavior change into those routines. For maximum success, the routines will have to be easy to use and have quick results. One immediate thing you can do is to begin adopting the second language of the common vernacular when speaking to your consumers (*reward* not reinforcement, *ignore* not extinction, etc.) followed by soliciting their input regarding goals, objectives, and preferred means of behavior change. If possible, you should try to include input from your consumers on the strategy for behavior change and prototype and test the behavior plan before it is cast in stone.

YOUNG PROFESSIONAL (3–5 YEARS)

Once you have had some experience with your own behavior analysis team implementing the elements of design thinking, you should have several success stories to share with the other behavior analysts in your organization. You may be able to train or supervise new BCBAs who come on board and are looking to try something new that they did not learn in grad school. Remember, you do not need to employ all the elements of this new approach but hopefully, you can adapt some of the ideas to different phases of your practice and make suggestions to newly trained behavior analysts.

MID-CAREER (6–10 YEARS)

By the time you are at mid-career, you will likely have some supervisory or administrative duties such as Director of Training or Clinical Director. In either of these posts, you are expected to recommend new processes and procedures that will improve the quality of care of your clients. You should be able to review the process for accepting new clients and use the *empathy* model in Step 1 to assure that your team of behavior analysts attends carefully to the needs of your parents and stakeholders right from the start of services. If you have been using design thinking for cases, you will by now probably have a roadmap of how this is done and can use this as a template for the services you provide. Putting an emphasis on Step 5, testing possible solutions to behavior problems before final implementation, is a sure way to demonstrate to your consumers that you are taking their needs into account and want to develop procedures that are custom-made for them with their input.

SENIOR BEHAVIOR ANALYST

As a senior behavior analyst, you are likely be a policy maker who is a CEO or member of the Board of Directors. One of your prime responsibilities is to assure that your company is not only fiscally successful but also viewed by the community as caring and responsible for quality treatment. Building an image for the public as a company that is innovative, responsive to clients, and very successful in the mission of humane, effective, behavior-change treatments will assure that the company will thrive in any competitive environment. Design thinking when used with every case will position your organization as competitive, flexible, and certainly client-centric.

SUMMARY

This chapter describes a method called *design thinking* that is widely used in business and industry to provide innovative solutions for customers. This *human-centric* approach puts the consumer at the center of the action using five steps: *empathize, define, ideate, prototype*, and *test*. The focus of design thinking on users (clients, stakeholders), their needs and motivation, is a good match for behavior analysis methodology. The emphasis on developing prototypes of behavior plans that can be tested to see if they are a good match for clients is another complimentary approach to ABA. At the end of a design thinking project, the consumer is asked if they were satisfied with the outcome. This is nearly identical to social validity measures that are often used in behavior analysis research. We recommend behavior analysts study the processes used in design thinking to improve their "products" (behavior-change programs) and their customers' (clients') satisfaction.

NOTE

1 For a larger project involving the analysis of a company's processes designers will include *systems thinking* (McKey, 2019), i.e., the interaction of several components of a larger unit, each element of which serves a different function.

REFERENCES

5 examples of design thinking in business. (n.d.). Retrieved from https://online.hbs.edu/blog/post/design-thinking-examples

8 great design thinking examples. (n.d). Retrieved from https://voltage-control.com/blog/8-great-design-thinking-examples/

Bailey, J. S., & Burch, M. R. (2018). *Research methods in applied behavior analysis* (2nd ed.). New York: Routledge, Inc.

Brandt, J. A., Dozier, C. L., Juanico, J. F., Laudont, C. L., & Mick, B. R. (2015). The value of choice as a reinforcer for typically developing children. *Journal of Applied Behavior Analysis, 48*, 344–362.

Brown, T. (2009). *Change by design: How design thinking transforms organizations and inspires innovation.* New York: HarperCollins Publishers.

Dam, R. F. (2022). *The 5 stages in the design thinking process.* Retrieved from www.interaction-design.org/literature/article/5-stages-in-the-design-thinking-process

Fisher, W. W., & Mazur, J. E. (1997). Basic and applied research on choice responding. *Journal of Applied Behavior Analysis, 48*, 387–410.

Hanratty, L. A., & Hanley, G. P. (2021). A preference analysis of reinforcer variation and choice. *Journal of Applied Behavior Analysis, 54*, 1062–1074.

Helvey, C. I., & Van Camp, C. M. (2022). Further comparison of isolated and synthesized contingencies in functional analysis. *Journal of Applied Behavior Analysis, 55*, 154–168.

Iwata, B. A., & Bailey, J. S. (1974). Reward versus cost token systems: An analysis of the effects on students and teacher. *Journal of Applied Behavior Analysis, 7*, 567–576.

Lewrick, M., Link, P., & Leifer, L. (2018). *The design thinking playbook: Mindful, digital transformation of teams, products, services, businesses, and ecosystems.* Hoboken, NJ: John Wiley & Sons, Inc.

McKey, Z. (2019). *Think in systems: The art of strategic planning, high efficiency problem-solving, and lasting results.* www.zoemckey.com.

Nava, M. J., Vargo, K. K., & Babino, M. M. (2016). An evaluation of a three-component multiple schedule to indicate attention availability. *Journal of Applied Behavior Analysis, 49*, 674–679. DOI: 10.1002/jaba.297

Pizarro, E. M., Vollmer, T. R., & Morris, S. L. (2021). Evaluating skills correlated with discriminated responding in multiple schedule arrangements. *Journal of Applied Behavior Analysis, 54*, 334–345.

Wolf, M. M. (1978). Social validity: The case for subjective measurement or how applied behavior analysis is finding its heart. *Journal of Applied Behavior Analysis, 11*, 203–214. https://doi.org/10.1901/jaba.1978.11-203

25

Aggressive Curiosity

I have no special talent. I am only passionately curious.

—Albert Einstein

You don't know what you don't know.

—Socrates

FRESH OUT OF GRAD SCHOOL, FIRST JOB

Children come into the world curious, asking questions about everything—"Why is the sky blue? Why does grandma cough all the time? Why can't we go to Disney World?"—but many their curiosity does not seem to maintain into adulthood. Something must have happened in their later education and family experiences where being inquisitive went on extinction or was punished. But there is a significant role for curiosity in science, the arts, business processes, *and* behavior analysis. We need people, lots of them, who are interested in human behavior and can exercise their curiosity every day as we seek answers to practical questions about our science and technology, our clients' actions, our therapists' skills, our caregivers' motivation, and possibly even our company's commitment to quality services for the vulnerable people in our charge.

DOI: 10.4324/9781003265573-30

A Personal Note from the First Author

Being *aggressively curious* means searching consistently and persistently for answers, digging deep into the topic, and diving into journal articles and reference works to get those questions answered.

I am fascinated with behavior and have been since my introduction to the topic in 1961 in Dr. Jack Michael's freshman course *Introduction to Behavior* at Arizona State University. Jack had a unique way of telling stories about his recent research in the pigeon lab (right down the hall from our classroom) and what it meant for understanding human behavior. His accounts of Dr. Ted Ayllon's work at a mental hospital in Saskatchewan, Canada, where Ted discovered the power of social reinforcement (delivered by nurses to shape behavior) captured my imagination. These were fascinating narratives of scientists making discoveries about how human behavior could be measured, carefully analyzed, and effectively modified. I was amazed to learn that behavior could be changed significantly by simply modifying the environment and that people's lives could be improved just by understanding the contingencies of reinforcement. This was a radical departure from traditional thinking that people acted the way they did because they *wanted to* or had some genetic trait that made them stubborn, aggressive, submissive, or manipulative. Jack Michael instilled in me a burning curiosity just by the colorful, enthusiastic way he described the settings and the people, and how he and Dr. Ayllon came up with ways to help them. Jack and Ted weren't working with much. They had B. F. Skinner's early books, *Walden Two*, *Science and Human Behavior*, *Verbal Behavior*, and a few volumes of the *Journal of the Experimental Analysis of Behavior*. But they were unencumbered by tradition, they were breaking new ground, and they knew it. Ayllon and Michael essentially created the field[1] with their *aggressive curiosity* about the relationship between behavior and environment. This desire to learn as much as I could about human behavior has lasted me a lifetime.

Being Aggressively *Curious*

Being curious from a behavioral perspective means searching consistently and persistently for answers, digging deep into the topic, and diving into journal articles and reference works to get those questions answered. Interesting, important questions regarding our clients and colleagues, stakeholders, CEOs, and our society are all around us. Even more broadly, questions appear in news headlines, public interviews with physicians, safety, and public health officials, and in documentaries on PBS and Netflix. There is a lot to learn about behavior, especially human behavior. It helps to have a schema that highlights relevant variables that may function to increase or decrease aggressive curiosity.

A Behavioral Analysis of Curiosity

When we are speaking of curious behavior as defined previously, it would be helpful to know what factors control such behavior since it is often lacking in adults. As a BCBA, you might be interested in encouraging some curious behaviors in your staff and even in your consumers. Figure 25.1 presents a diagram of variables that seem to be relevant. *Setting events* are environmental events that do not produce any specific behavior but can motivate a person to engage in a class of behavior that would not normally be seen. Being suddenly let go from a job, a death in the family, or winning a lottery might set the occasion for classes of responses ranging from desperate to extravagant. *Antecedents* are well known as stimuli specifically designed to elicit a particular response; one frequently used stimulus is a *brainstorming* session (described in Chapter 24). The *person* in Figure 25.1 is where the history of reinforcement resides and their current biological condition

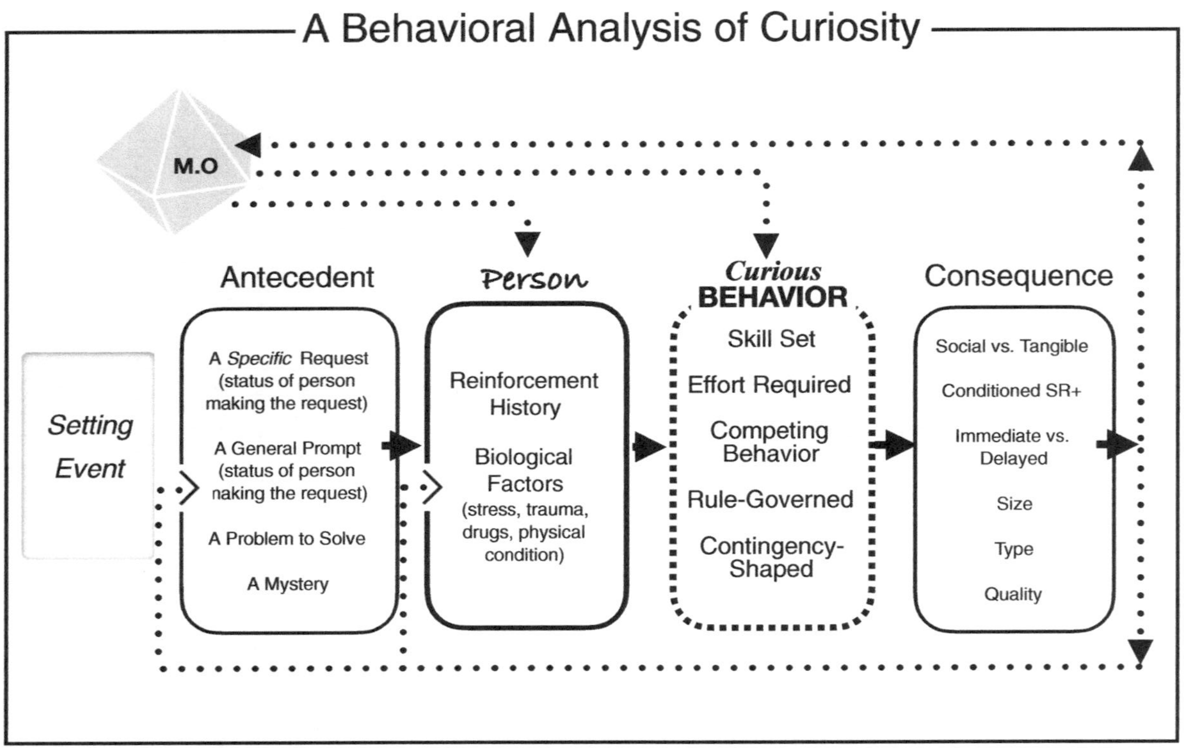

Figure 25.1 This graphic illustrates some likely controlling variables for curiosity.

(e.g., tired, stressed, medicated, sleep deprived) is accounted for including the possibility of a trauma history; to encourage creative responding we want our participants to be well rested and relaxed. Certain deprivation conditions and aversive situations can directly affect the motivation of a person to engage in certain classes of behavior; we call these *MOs*. At the end of this string of events and conditions, a behavior is emitted and if we are trying to produce *curious behavior* all those earlier events will have been designed precisely to produce this behavior. The behavior analyst working to get their team thinking creatively will need to provide *consequences* that are highly reinforcing for new ideas, new lines of inquiry, and thinking-out-of-the-box solutions.

Some Tips on Boosting Your Own Aggressive Curiosity

One way to increase your curiosity is to contact other professionals via state, national, even international conferences. You need a lot of stimulation, many things to think about and ponder, and issues to connect to activate your curiosity. Are there advances in medicine or strategies being used in rehabilitation that might relate to a problem you are working on? How did they come up with this idea? Why do they deal with their problem in this way? You might find yourself saying, "If they hired me, here's what I would do to solve that problem." If you do this routinely and get into the habit of talking back to your computer monitor or TV screen, you'll find that ideas jump out that relate to a problem you're having right now in your organization or with a client. While working out, driving to work, or waiting for your next flight, consider listening to a *Curiosity Podcast*. There are dozens of them on a wide range of topics to stimulate your interest and encourage curiosity. Follow up with some aggressive curiosity and you are on your way.

Keep a Notebookw

You may come up with ideas throughout the week based on something you heard on National Public Radio (NPR), have read on

Google or Apple News, or picked up in a conversation. If it is new or strikes you as unusual or funny, write it down and indicate the date and where you heard the idea so you can track it down later. The first author keeps his iPhone handy in his car and will pull off the road to dictate a note about a news story or an interview. A few years ago, *All Things Considered* (NPR) featured an interview with Amy Sutherland, the best-selling author of *Kicked, Bitten, and Scratched* (2006). This led to tracking down her agent and eventually a phone call with the author herself in which she was invited to give the keynote address at the annual meeting of the Florida Association for Behavior Analysis. She stimulated the thinking of nearly a thousand behavior analysts with her address based on her recent book *What Shamu Taught Me About Life, Love, and Marriage* (2008).

Watch Indie Films

The blockbuster films that occupy 90% of the screens in America don't often provide us with food for thought, but documentaries and independent films do. Often made on low budgets by creative people with a unique perspective on the world, these films portray human behavior in all its vast and glorious diversity. They capture human behavior under circumstances we could never imagine and challenge us to understand how and why people do what they do.

Meet New People

If you have a regular posse and do everything together, you will soon begin to think in such uniform terms that you'll begin finishing each other's sentences. Every now and then, consider making a new friend from a different line of work or a different religion or culture. Use this as an opportunity to see how this person reacts to challenges you have and learn how your new friend would deal with your challenges. This can be stimulating and invigorating and may take you in directions you never imagined.

Question Conventional Wisdom

The commercial culture in which we live has a powerful interest in getting you to operate as a consumer in standard, conventional ways without thinking about what you are doing or why. Be prepared to challenge this from time to time at work and in your personal life. Use caution, however, when it comes to challenging work-related issues unless you're sure you have a much better solution than what is being done now.

Ask the Function Question

Our culture brainwashes us into accepting standard solutions to common problems, and it is easy to get in a rut of conventional thinking. As a behavior analyst, you are trained to ask about the function of behavior. Now ask that same question about larger issues you must deal with every day. Parents ask for help with their children's disruptive, out-of-control behavior; shouldn't we ask ourselves how this happened and why? Schools use suspension as a punisher, but it doesn't appear to work. What are the alternatives? We usually get paid by the hour, but shouldn't we really be paid instead for the results we achieve? Why the focus in functional analysis on *Demand* contingencies? Rather than using escape extinction to essentially force the client to comply with a "demand" why not just modify the question? Make it an *ask* not a *demand* and make it interesting for clients to respond.

Challenge the Status Quo

The test of aggressive curiosity is whether you can make a difference with a new idea you've discovered. Digging deeper for an answer, saying "no" to a conventional proposal, bringing a new person or new perspective to the table, and pushing it hard will make you and others uncomfortable, but it is probably a good sign that you are on to something. You are respecting your business client if you learn everything you can about the history of the company, have memorized the table of organization, and have read the annual reports for the past five years. In a recent consultation, we were asked to figure out what it would take to get computer hardware sales associates to push software add-ons. It didn't take long to determine that the company had long-standing incentives for hardware sales but none for software. It had never occurred to the company managers that it was this absence of an incentive that was the issue, not laziness or stubbornness on the part of the associates. The company managers were locked into a theory of behavior that we were able to challenge, and we could see the furrowed brows of "Why didn't we think of that?" on their faces.

Behaviorally Related Topics to Explore With Aggressive Curiosity

Virtual and Augmented Reality

Virtual reality (VR) is used now in video games, sports, medicine, and education[2] and there is no reason that it will not become a significant part of behavior analysis and therapy. If VR could be used to teach doctors to perform brain surgery or gymnasts to perform elaborate floor routines, then surely we could use it to teach interview-informed synthesized contingency analysis, how to conduct complex assessments and interviews, and learn about other cultures. By creating computer-generated artificial environments, we could more rapidly and thoroughly train RBTs, and with advances in applications of behavioral research, there could be developed a library of treatments for a variety of specialty areas including pica, eating disorders, SIB, sexual dysfunction, and more. Rather than having to bring in experts to consult or conduct the training, they could send a set of VR videos that could be used as needed. The state of this technology has been reviewed (Turnacioglu, McGleery, Parish-Morris, Sazawal, & Solorzano, 2019) and single-case design research with ASD clients is underway (E. Ingvarsson, personal communication, July 28, 2022) using an AR device by Floreo[3] invented by Sinan Turnacioglu, MD, which is showing quite promising data. The Floreo device is currently available on a monthly subscription basis.

Augmented Reality (AR) is similar except that it takes the existing environment and inserts artificial images that the person can respond to—think desensitization to a fear of dogs or closed spaces, for example.

TAGteach

Clicker training has been used for years in animal training and has been adapted to teaching complex human performances by dancers (Quinn, Miltenberger, & Fogel, 2015, #48), golfers (Fogel, Weil, & Burris, 2010), rugby players (Elmore, Healy, Lydon, & Murray, 2018), and yoga students (Ennett, Zonneveld, Thomson, Vause, & Ditor, 2020). This seems like a very promising approach to use in clinical and community settings with a wide variety of motor behaviors for a range of clients from pre-school to adults.

Adverse Childhood Experiences (ACEs) aka Trauma

Behavior analysis may be late to the game of recognizing the profound effect that ACEs can have on children (Rajaraman et al., 2022) but this is an area of treatment that needs exploration, aggressive curiosity about how to detect early signs of trauma, and of course, the effective treatment of these behaviors could be a critical new area for our field.

YOUNG PROFESSIONAL (3–5 YEARS)

Assuming you have been successful in enhancing your own aggressive curiosity repertoire and that of your immediate staff of RBTs and trainees, at this stage of your career you may be able to expand your influence to other BCBAs at your company or clinic. With numerous examples of new treatment strategies you have discovered or developed, you should be able to give in-house presentations on "Promoting Aggressive Curiosity" by filling out the schema shown in Figure 25.2.

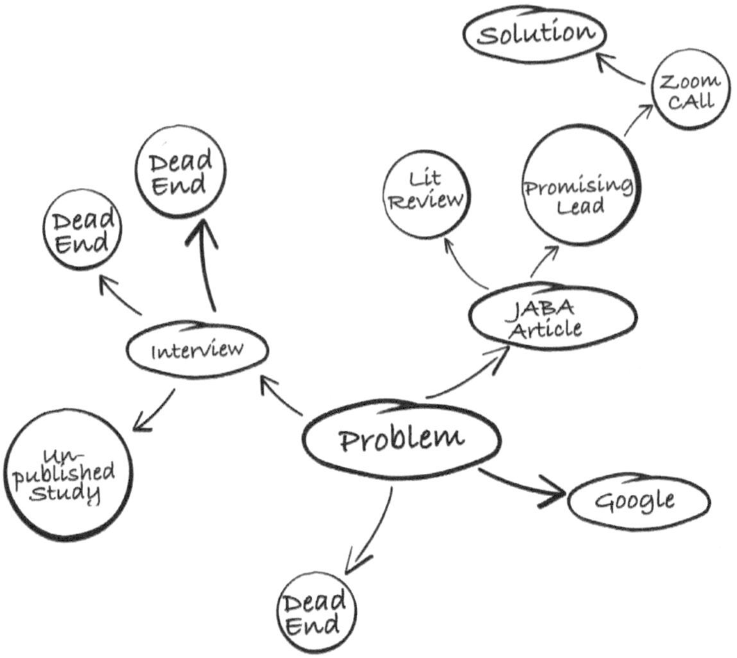

Figure 25.2 Aggressive curiosity often produces dead ends and usually involves several stages of inquiry before new answers and solutions emerge.

MID-CAREER (6–10 YEARS)

With years of experience in helping others expand their curiosity about the world, this is the time to share your discoveries with a broader audience. Learning how nature and the built environment work makes a person more fully appreciate the complexity of our domain and enriches our thinking and appreciation for the dedication of those around us. At mid-career, you should have a satisfying and rich repertoire of ideas and knowledge that will give you the confidence to lead those around you to adopt an aggressive curiosity lifestyle.

SENIOR BEHAVIOR ANALYST

Since you will likely be in upper management, at this point you will have ample opportunity to encourage aggressive curiosity about all manner of issues that come to your attention from how to: attract talented behavior analysts in your company and retain them, create a strong corporate culture, manage company finances, keep up with behavioral technology, satisfy clients and consumers, and produce high-quality behavior-change that makes a lasting difference.

SUMMARY

This chapter presents the need for behavior analysts to become aggressively curious about all manner of topics related to our field. Being *aggressively curious* means searching consistently and persistently for answers, digging deep into the topic, and diving into journal articles and reference works to get those questions answered. A behavioral analysis of the controlling variables that enhance or discourage curiosity is presented and examples are given of how you can use this knowledge to increase curiosity on the part of your staff. Tips are provided on how to increase your own aggressive curiosity by keeping a notebook of ideas and questions that come up from day to day, making a habit of watching indie films and documentaries, meeting new people, questioning conventional wisdom, asking the function question, and challenging the status quo.

NOTES

1 Ayllon, T., & Michael, J. (1959). The psychiatric nurse as a behavioral engineer. *Journal of the Experimental Analysis of Behavior*, *2*, 323–334.
2 www.iberdrola.com/innovation/virtual-reality
3 www.floreotech.com

FOR FURTHER READING

Berger, W. (2019). *The book of beautiful questions: The powerful questions that will help you decide, create, connect, and lead*. New York: Bloomsbury Publishing.

Ennett, T. M., Zonneveld, K. L. M., Thomson, K. M., Vause, T., & Ditor, D. (2020). Comparison of two TAGteach error-correction procedures to teach beginner yoga poses to adults. *Journal of Applied Behavior Analysis*, *53*(1), 222–236. https://doi.org/10.1002/jaba.550

Hamilton, D. (2018). *Cracking the curiosity code: The key to unlocking human potential.* Columbus, OH: Gatekeeper Press.

Taberner, K., & Siggins, K. T. (2015). *The power of curiosity: How to have real conversations that create collaboration, innovation and understanding.* New York: Morgan James Publishing.

REFERENCES

Ayllon, T., & Michael, J. (1959). The psychiatric nurse as a behavioral engineer. *Journal of the Experimental Analysis of Behavior, 2,* 323–334.

Elmore, T., Healy, O., Lydon, S., & Murray, C. (2018). An evaluation of teaching with acoustical guidance (TAGteach) for improving passing skills among university rugby athletes. *Journal of Sport Behavior, 41*(4).

Fogel, V. A., Weil, T. M., & Burris, H. (2010). Evaluating the efficacy of TAGteach as a training strategy for teaching a golf swing. *Journal of Behavioral Health and Medicine, 1*(1), 25–41. https://doi.org/10.1037/h0100539

Quinn, M. J., Miltenberger, R. G., & Fogel, V. A. (2015). Using TAGteach to improve the proficiency of dance movements. *Journal of Applied Behavior Analysis, 48*(1), 11–24.

Rajaraman, A., Austin, J. L., Gover, H. C., Cammilleri, A. P., Donnely, D. R., & Hanley, G. P. (2022). Toward trauma-informed applications of behavior analysis. *Journal of Applied Behavior Analysis, 55*(1), 40–61. http://doi.org/10.1002/jaba.881. Epub 2021 September 15.

Sutherland, A. (2006). *Kicked, bitten, and scratched: Life lessons at the world's premier school for exotic animal trainers.* New York: Penguin Books.

Sutherland, A. (2008). *What Shamu taught me about life, love, and marriage: Lessons for people from animals and their trainers.* New York: Random House.

Turnacioglu, S., McGleery, J. P., Parish-Morris, J., Sazawal, V., & Solorzano, R. (2019). The state of virtual and augmented reality therapy for autism spectrum disorder (ASD). In G. Guazzaroni (Ed.), *Virtual and augmented reality in mental health* (pp. 118–140). GI Global.

About the Authors

Jon S. Bailey received his PhD from the University of Kansas in 1970 and is *Professor Emeritus* of *Psychology* at Florida State University where he was on the graduate faculty for 38 years and produced a record 63 PhDs. He is currently on the faculty of the FSU Panama City master's program in Psychology with a specialty in Applied Behavior Analysis and teaches Ethics & Professional Issues, Skinner's Theory of Behaviorism, and Research Methods in ABA.

He is a Board Certified Behavior Analyst; is a Fellow of the Association for Behavior Analysis: International and the American Psychological Association; he is Secretary/Treasurer, Program Co-Chair, and Media Coordinator for the Florida Association for Behavior Analysis, which he founded in 1980.

Dr. Bailey has published over 100 peer-reviewed research articles, is past-Editor of the *Journal of Applied Behavior Analysis* and is co-author/editor of 18 books including: *Research Methods in Applied Behavior Analysis, How Dogs Learn, Ethics for Behavior Analysts, How to Think Like a Behavior Analyst, 25 Essential Skills and Strategies for Professional Behavior Analysts, Ethics for Behavior Analysts, 2nd Expanded* Edition and *Ethics for Behavior Analysts*, 3rd and 4th Editions; most were co-authored with Dr. Mary R. Burch. One additional book is *Performance Management: Changing Behavior that Drives Organizational Effectiveness*, with Dr. Aubrey Daniels, which was published in 2014. *Research Methods in Applied Behavior Analysis*, 2nd Edition was published in 2018; *How to Think Like a Behavior Analyst* published in 2022.

Dr. Bailey received the **Distinguished Service to Behavior Analysis Award**, May 2005, from the Society for the Advancement of Behavior Analysis, both the APA Division 25, **Fred S. Keller Behavioral Education Award** and the University of Kansas **Applied Behavioral Science Distinguished Alumni Award** in 2012. He served on the Board of Directors of Goodwill Industries Big Bend for the past five years. He received the prestigious **Nathan H. Azrin Award for Outstanding Contributions to Applied Behavior Analysis** from the American Psychological Association in August 2014 and received a Lifetime Achievement Award from the Florida Association for Behavior Analysis in 2020.

Mary R. Burch, PhD, is a Board Certified Behavior Analyst™ (BCBA-D). She is also a Certified Applied Animal Behaviorist. Dr. Burch has authored or co-authored 20 books. She is an award-winning writer whose work has appeared in books, magazines, syndicated newspaper columns and on radio. Her behavioral research has been published by the U.S. Department of Education. Dr. Burch has developed online training courses for behavior analysts on topics such as Ethics and Supervision, and she has co-authored several best-selling books in the field of behavior analysis.

Index